Managing Managed Care

Clinical Child Psychology Library

Series Editors: Michael C. Roberts and Annette M. La Greca

A Continuation Order Plan is available for this series. A continuation order will bring delivery
of each new volume immediately upon publication. Volumes are billed only upon actual
shipment. For further information please contact the publisher.

Managing Managed Care

Michael C. Roberts
University of Kansas
Lawrence, Kansas

and

Linda K. Hurley
Private Practice
Fort Worth, Texas

Plenum Press • New York and London

Library of Congress Cataloging-in-Publication Data

Roberts, Michael C.
    Managing managed care / Michael C. Roberts and Linda K. Hurley.
        p.   cm. -- (Clinical child psychology library)
    Includes bibliographical references and index.
    ISBN 0-306-45670-2 (hbk.). -- ISBN 0-306-45671-0 (pbk.)
    1. Managed mental health care.   I. Hurley, Linda K.   II. Title.
III. Series.
RC465.5.R63 1997
362.2'0425--dc21   97-33280
                                                                   CIP

RC 465.5 .R63 1997

Roberts, Michael C.

Managing managed care

ISBN 0-306-45670-2 (Hardbound)
ISBN 0-306-45671-0 (Paperback)

© 1997 Plenum Press, New York
A Division of Plenum Publishing Corporation
233 Spring Street, New York, N. Y. 10013

http://www.plenum.com

10 9 8 7 6 5 4 3 2 1

Printed in the United States of America

To our mentors,
for opening the world of psychology to us and helping us to know
ourselves better

Preface

The introduction of the concept of managed care into mental and physical health care appears to be a juggernaut of unparalleled impact. The two extremes of thought about this impact are (1) that managed care is a villainous foe to be resisted in order to bring back the earlier halcyon years of independence in practice decisions with greater reimbursement for psychologists' services or (2) that managed care is a laudatory attempt to restrain health care costs that are out of control and spiraling upward by rooting out mismanagement and reversing financial incentives to provide unnecessary care. The former view calls managed health care such names as "mangled care" and distributes bumper stickers stating "Just Say No to HMOs." The latter view points to the slowdown of increases in health care expenditures and the enhancement of health care affordability and appropriateness for greater numbers of persons resulting from managed care cost-containment strategies and service review procedures.

Mental or behavioral health care has been as strongly impacted as medical care under managed care. Where managed care has forced practitioners' attention to validated procedures and to examining previous wasteful practices, we applaud the movement. Where managed care has had adverse impact, we think there needs to be greater public, legal, and regulatory attention to its excesses and abuses. What is needed for behavioral health care is the equivalent of a public outcry over "drive-by deliveries" and "outpatient mastectomies" to focus on fulfilling the need for quality and accessible behavioral health care services while maintaining appropriate accountability from mental health professionals. We believe policy advocacy needs to focus on the failure to provide adequate services for children, adolescents, and families in the private and public sectors. This aspect has, so far, been largely neglected in the efforts of major professional organizations. Child-oriented clinicians will need to address individually and collectively how these campaigns are formulated.

In this volume, we provide information useful to the clinician who seeks to work within a managed care environment as well as the clinician who wishes to remain outside it or to have limited involvement with managed care organizations. In the following chapters, we tried to avoid the problems conveyed by the acronym COIK—"clear only if known"—so that one does not have to be well-versed in managed care concepts in order to use the volume. Similarly, we wanted to avoid providing such overly basic information that the more experienced clinician would not find the discussion useful.

We envisioned the purposes of this volume as fivefold. We intend that it will:

1	Inform the clinician (especially the clinical child/pediatric psychologist) about the managed care system: what types of managed care systems exist, how they work, and what the advantages and pitfalls of working within these systems are.
2	Assist the clinician in providing quality and effective services to children and their families within the managed care system.
3	Help the clinician understand how to work within the managed care system without being significantly harmed financially, legally, or professionally.
4	Help the clinician identify other ways of practicing without entering the managed care system or of restricting the percentage of their practice that is based on managed care.
5	Provide information for trainers and students about the managed care environment with special applications to the issues of children, adolescents, and families.

We have organized the book into seven chapters with attention to the basics of managed care, the problems posed by managed care, legal and ethical issues for the clinician in managed care, adapting to the managed care environment, limiting negative impact of managed care on a clinical child/pediatric psychology practice, practicing outside managed care, and the scientific bases for clinical practice.

We thank series editor Annette La Greca for her editorial comments and Noel Jacobs, Jodi Kamps, Regina Kinney, Dawn Koontz, Cecilia Robertson, and Brenda Spreier Rump for their helpful markings on an earlier version. Our professional colleagues in the clinical child and pediatric psychology specialty also helped shape this book.

Michael C. Roberts
Linda K. Hurley

Contents

Basics of Managed Care in Psychological Services for Children and Families

A psychologist, "fed up" with delayed payments and externally imposed limits on what he could do professionally for his clients in assessment and psychotherapy, removed himself from all managed care panels. He set up consulting arrangements with group homes and local daycare centers and developed a self-pay market. He negotiated a contract with a local philanthropic organization to do evaluations/interventions with children living at the organization-sponsored home for battered women. Although he faced some short-term loss of income and long-term changes in what he did hour to hour, he found the new practice financially and psychologically rewarding.

A psychologist in independent practice of 20 years specializing in eating disorders was told by a clerk for a managed care company (with a B.A. in sociology) that her review of the case record indicated that treatment beyond six sessions for an anoretic client was unnecessary according to the treatment protocol book. The clinician wrote a formal appeal of the decision, citing the relevant clinical research literature and indicating that, once the sixth session was completed, responsibility for the welfare of the client would necessarily return to the managed care organization. A copy of this letter was given to the client's parents, who raised concerns with the employer's benefits office.

A married couple, both licensed psychologists, were in practice together. They aligned themselves with one managed care company and relied heavily on that health maintenance organization (HMO) for their patients. They felt they had an excellent relationship with the HMO, and the HMO seemed pleased with their work as they continued to refer

> many patients to the practice. The HMO suddenly decided to contract directly with a psychiatric hospital to provide all their mental health services and dropped the two psychologists with very short notice. They lost their practice because they had too few patients to pay the bills after that particular HMO ceased doing business with them.

Health care in the United States, including both physical and mental health services, has developed into an enormously expensive proposition. As a result of increasing health care expenses, numerous schemes have been proposed and implemented through the years to control costs. The latest, and perhaps most powerful, scheme to develop has been subsumed under the label "managed care." As reflected in the vignettes opening this chapter, nothing has altered so dramatically the practice of psychology, as well as other mental health and medical care fields, as the managed care "revolution." What is this revolutionary catalyst of change? Like many revolutions, managed care philosophy derives from relatively simple concepts. Managed care is a composite term for the attempts by those who organize or pay for health care services to control the costs of those services, presumably without a loss in quality or effectiveness.

This cost-control comes about in several ways. First and foremost, advocates for managed care principles argue that costs are reduced by eliminating unnecessary services (i.e., those parts of health care that are not proven effective or not demonstrably needed). Second, costs are further reduced by contracting with care providers for reduced fee reimbursement (i.e., contracting with the "lowest bidder" for nominally similar services). Third, cost savings are gained by restricting coverage to certain categories of diagnoses or treatments and not extending coverage to others (i.e., excluding reimbursement for treatment of certain problems or conditions). Fourth, managed care operations attempt to control costs by placing limits or parameters on how the treatment is actually conducted (e.g., through limits imposed on the number of sessions to be reimbursed or reimbursement only for certain, specific types of treatment). These and other changes in contracting and payment for health care are discussed throughout this volume as we outline ways for the clinician to manage managed care.

Throughout our discussion, we recognize that the various parties in a health care relationship often have different needs and purposes that conflict in the accessing of services (consumers), the provision of services (clinicians), the reimbursement for those services (insurance companies), and the purchasing of the reimbursement plans (employers). At this point in the United States the key power is seemingly held in the purchasing and reimbursement practices for health care services, and less power is held by those accessing and providing the services. The business orientation of managed care has been succinctly articulated as: "For-profit HMOs owe, by law, first allegiance to their shareholders. Their employer-customers are second on the queue, patients a distant third" (Woolhandler & Himmelstein, 1996, p. 1699). By business criteria, these arrangements have been successful. For example, in January 1997, the Associated Press reported that "HMOs and other managed-care plans have helped contain health insurance inflation for the third consecutive year, according to a widely watched survey" ("Health Insurance Inflation Stays Low," 1997, p. D-6). Indeed, the stocks of managed care companies have been excellent investments, although this profitable trend may change because there may be fewer ways to cut costs and turn over profits. Also importantly, changes in procedures will be compelled by public and professional demands for quality, accessible care. Regulation and the threat of regulation will also effect some changes. While managed care has several advantages, there are inevitably a multitude of disadvantages (as there were with all previous forms of health care financing). The conflicts usually can be reduced to those regarding controlling costs. Indeed, with the emphasis on costs in the managed care revolution, several commentators have noted that the term "managed costs" is more appropriate because "care" is nowhere apparent in the discussion.

CHANGES IN THINKING ABOUT HEALTH CARE REIMBURSEMENT

Americans' attitudes toward and thoughts about health care have changed dramatically over the past decade or so. People generally expect far more from their health insurance than before. The push toward preventive health care services has somehow been transformed into an attitude of "I should receive every service available at no cost to me." Clearly, this cannot actually happen. Just for comparison, let us contrast auto insurance with health care insurance. Traditionally, indemnity-type health insurance was designed to cover the expenses associated with catastrophic illness or injury: a heart attack, cancer, or injuries from an automobile wreck. The consumer (or more often an individual's employer) paid a premium to the insurer to cover those costs in the unlikely event the catastrophe occurred and the services were needed. Other health care costs, such as for routine physical exams, blood work, and others, were paid from the consumer's pocket.

Automobile insurance worked in much the same way. Auto insurance covered relatively unlikely occurrences such as a wreck, hail damage, or injury to a passenger caused by the insured driver's behavior. Now what if automobile insurance had changed in the same way health insurance has changed? People would expect their insurance to cover oil changes, new tires, and other routine maintenance expenses along with those unexpected catastrophes mentioned here. Would it be possible for an automobile insurance company to provide all those services for the same premium as it charged for just the catastrophes? Not likely. What would probably happen is that the insurance company would need to impose restrictions on what things were actually covered: an individual can only get one oil change every 6 months, even if the car is driven 3000 miles per month. If a person drives that much, the driver is on his or her own to cover more frequent oil changes—that is not a "covered benefit." If the driver wants to go to a personally chosen mechanic (a trusted and competent one), the driver would have to pay for that out of pocket, because the auto insurance company has contracted with one business, "Bubba's Speedy Lube," to do oil changes for $7 each (Bubba tries to make a profit in the volume of business or cuts his own business costs and standard of living). The insurance company is not about to pay $29.95 for service at the insured's personal mechanic. Similarly, hail damage (except for broken glass) would not affect a car's performance or a person's ability to drive the car, even though it may not look very good. Therefore, hail damage repair, in this comparison, would not be a "medically necessary" condition, and the insurance company would likely no longer pay for it. As can be seen, the car insurance company has to look for more ways to cut costs, either by contracting for discounted service, by reducing the types of services available, or by placing obstacles in the way of those who seek to receive the covered services.

This scenario illustrates what has happened in health care. By demanding that all services be covered by their health insurance policies, consumers have forced changes in the structure of health reimbursement systems. This has resulted in cheaper services (and reduced reimbursement for providers), limitations on types of health services available, and obstacles to accessing services. Additionally, the obstacles and limitations are often hidden from the consumer until a need for those benefits arises.

CHANGES AFFECTING PSYCHOLOGICAL PRACTICES

For psychologists and other mental health providers, the managed care movement has resulted in significant changes in the way their services are provided and reimbursed from the way they were just a few years ago. These changes include restrictions on clinicians in making treatment decisions, whereas they were previously unrestricted in the length, form, or content of psychotherapy. Independent practitioners are now more likely to enter into group practices than in the past. They are doing more consulting and less traditional independent practice (assessment and individual therapy) than previously. Independent practitioners are becoming very creative in finding niche markets for their services. Inpatient providers have changed from doing evaluation, diagnosis, and trial treatment to purely crisis stabilization, and length of stays have dropped dramatically, often inappropriately. Horror stories are frequently told such as the suicidal patient discharged after 3 days of 24-hour-a-day watch who then reattempted suicide after being home for a few hours. The managed care company justified the discharge, stating that the patient had not attempted suicide in the 3 days in the hospital. School psychologists are also feeling overwhelmed as parents try to find some place to have their children evaluated for problems like attention-deficit hyperactivity disorder (ADHD), which their insurance no longer covers.

A 1996 survey of psychologists by the American Psychological Association's (APA's) Committee for the Advancement of Professional Practice (CAPP) revealed that fewer psychologists are entering independent practice now than at any previous time (APA Practice Directorate, 1996; "Practitioner Survey Results," 1996). It appears that market forces are driving newly licensed practitioners into practice with groups and larger systems and to academic and government jobs. In fact, more psychologists licensed between 1990 and 1995 entered the work force in medical settings than ever before. The solo independent practitioner remained the dominant form of practice from 1990–1995, but at a lower level than in prior years.

Why might this be? According to survey results, psychologists report that managed care is changing clinical practice and is presenting many more ethical dilemmas than ever before. Practitioners cited excess concerns with precertification and utilization review (UR) requirements of managed care panels and decreased income because of managed care fee reductions. In fact, 80% of those responding to the survey stated that managed care had a negative impact on their professional work, and those in independent practice indicated the most negative impact of all. Over all settings, 48% of psychologists reported income reduction because of decreased fees through managed care, with 62% of those in solo practice and 73% of those in group practices endorsing that concern. Although managed care companies generally promise an increase in patients as a benefit of doing business with them, 40% of all psychologists surveyed (52% of those in solo practice and 42% of those in group practices) indicated they had fewer patients because of managed care. Overall, 49% of psychologists stated that excessive UR and precertification was a problem and that the amount of increase in paperwork was significant; practicing psychologists reported that they spend about 13% of their time doing administrative tasks, including UR and clinical documentation.

According to a survey of subscribers to *Behavior Today*, 86% believe that quality of mental health care suffers when provided in a managed care system ("*BT* Survey Results," July 20, 1987; Newman & Bricklin, 1991). The majority of complaints were similar to the CAPP survey and were related to caps on the number of sessions allowed, increased paperwork, and the gate-keeper system, with additional complaints about lack of flexibility in treatment approaches allowed, delayed reimbursement by the third-party payer, and use of nonpsychologists as gatekeepers. However, there may be some advantages to involvement in a managed care system. Some of those cited in the *Behavior Today* survey include increased patient flow, less marketing needed by providers, increased income, and general economic benefits, albeit at the expense of quality of care.

Psychologists and other mental health providers rail against the managed care juggernaut and lament over the changes from the halcyon years of fee-for-service insurance reimbursement with few strings attached. Different commentators have advanced various arguments supporting anti-managed care positions, yet sometimes these arguments conflict, even for those opposed to managed care. At times psychologists, in particular, have been their most vocal critics. Some argue that psychological assessment and treatment is only competent from highly trained doctoral level practitioners, whereas others point to research that less well-trained mental health workers are equally effective. Some advance the notion of psychology as "behavioral health" rather than mental health in order to ally with some health maintenance orientations; others debate the merits of mental health "carve-outs." Some argue that "medical cost offsets" prove the value of psychological interventions in the managed care system. Others argue that medical offset savings from mental health treatment are illusory. Some argue for only "empirically based" interventions for reimbursement, while others find the evidence lacking for one treatment approach above another (even suggesting that, in the absence of compelling data, nobody should get reimbursement unless everybody is eligible). Some argue that managed care is here to stay and psychological practitioners had better get used to it. Others have advocated a return to the years of unrestricted reimbursement for psychotherapy. Yet others point to the past with its professional hubris and lack of scrutiny, even fraud, when almost anything was acceptable, arguing that closer cost management was inevitable, even laudable.

Some argue for an acceptance of a newly emerging status quo; others argue that resistance, even subterfuge or manipulation, of managed care is necessary to undermine it. Thus, a great deal of verbiage has been expended as the penetration of managed care into mental health benefits and practice has increased over time. Surely these arguments serve to confuse the situation, but all points need to be presented and scrutinized. In all our reading and listening, rarely has any statement from anybody been totally without some kernel of truth. We hope to present a balanced view, helpful to the practitioner and informative to the trainer and student.

THE ABCs OF MANAGED CARE

The variations within the insurance industry today look like alphabet soup: Everything seems to have an acronym. There are basically three major forms of health insurance available today: Health maintenance organizations (HMOs), preferred provider organizations (PPOs), and major medical or indemnity plans. Although there are many other acronyms in use for variations on these plans and in reference to provider group types, these three form the backbone of the industry.

HMOs

HMOs are legal entities, licensed by the state department of health or state department of insurance, that combine the insurance of health care with the delivery of health care services. HMOs charge a fixed fee to prepay health care costs, and then arrange for the delivery of health care to enrollees through a prearranged system. By law (the HMO Act of 1973), HMOs must have these four characteristics: (1) an organized system for providing health care in a geographic region, (2) an agreed-upon set of basic and supplemental health maintenance and treatment services, (3) a voluntarily enrolled group of subscribers, and (4) community rating. Community rating means that payment rates must be fixed so that they are equivalent for all individuals and for all families of similar composition. The purpose of community rating is to spread the cost of health care evenly over all subscribers rather than charging more to sick people.

HMOs were originally intended to increase access to health care for preventive care by decreasing fee-for-service disincentives. When they were shown to be cost-effective, they were expanded to cover older and sicker patients who were more costly. Over the past several years, HMOs have abandoned their social objectives in favor of economic ones. The emphasis in HMOs is on limiting the supply of services, often by managing providers and their behavior. HMOs use UR (utilization review) to limit use to below what is offered as covered benefits. There are special threats to mental health from managed care, such as discriminatory coverage for substance abuse and mental disorders by such mechanisms as preexisting conditions (Dorwart, 1990). Many plans expressly exclude conduct/behavioral disorders and developmental, learning, and attention problems. Some plans exclude marriage, family, or child counseling.

The federal HMO Act of 1973 only requires HMOs to offer limited mental health services, including only short-term outpatient services that cannot exceed 20 outpatient mental health visits per year under basic (not supplemental) benefits. Inpatient mental health care is not considered a basic benefit, although it may be offered, at the HMO's choice, as a supplemental health service. There is a difference in requirements between HMOs that are federally qualified (by participating in the Medicare program) and those that are not. Medicare participants are regulated by federal law, which preempts state HMO laws. Some states provide mandatory mental health coverage under their "basic health care services" provisions, whereas others do not. HMOs often are not required by state law to include mental health and drug/alcohol abuse services in their basic health care services. In addition, the definition of "health care provider/ professional" varies from state to state. The clinician must check the state's laws for applicable rules. State and federal laws and regulations are constantly changing, so the clinician is best advised to stay informed through state associations and practice groups.

The parity amendment to the 1997 appropriations legislation for Veterans Affairs/Housing and Urban Development, effective in January 1998, mandates parity (or equality) of mental health and medical benefits in terms of dollar maximums (Sleek, 1996d). For example, if a policy has a lifetime medical benefit maximum of $1 million, it would have to include mental health benefits under that same maximum or offer the same dollar amount of coverage for mental health. The law, which applies to all group health plans covering 50 or more beneficiaries, also pertains to self-insured plans, which have previously been exempt from most government legislation. However, companies may still restrict the number of visits per year, and may impose other restrictions on access to mental health services.

HMOs present an inherent conflict of interest because of the fact that the insurer is also the provider of services. Most states require evidence of financial health of the HMO and a guarantee that the HMO will be able to perform its obligations to the enrollees.

Within HMOs, there are several subtypes:

1	Staff model: An HMO that delivers health services through a salaried provider group employed by the HMO.
2	Group model: An HMO that contracts with an independent group practice to deliver health care services.
3	Network: An HMO that contracts with two or more independent group practices, possibly including a staff group, or solo practitioners to provide health care services.
4	Independent practice associations (IPAs): Individuals or small groups of providers that form a larger group for the purpose of contracting with managed care organizations, often to receive capitated contracts.
5	Open-ended HMOs: These are more like PPOs in that enrollees are covered, by their choice and without referral, to receive services outside of the HMO network. Coverage is similar to that in a traditional major medical plan and is available at any time. Benefits

are generally less comprehensive outside the network and usually include deductibles, copayments, and/or coinsurance.

6   Capitation plans: Capitation is an arrangement where a group of providers is paid a fixed fee for each patient enrolled regardless of the number or type of services provided. The patient generally must identify the provider as his or her chosen provider, but payment may sometimes be withheld until or unless the patient actually accesses services the first time.

7   Point of service (POS) options: HMOs that offer POS options allow consumers to go outside the plan for specified care. The consumer pays a considerably higher copayment/deductible, but has a wider choice of providers. Inpatient services and surgeries must still be precertified. Several states are currently considering or have passed legislation making POS mandatory and are limiting the out-of-pocket charges the consumer must pay.

PPOs

PPOs are health care financing and delivery programs that provide financial incentives to consumers who utilize a "preferred" group of health care providers. Providers typically receive discounted fee payment on a fee-for-service basis in exchange for the PPO's promise of increased patient volume and quick reimbursement. Consumers generally have a choice of providers, but receive financial incentives through smaller copayments or lower deductibles to choose those on the PPO panel.

PPOs may be exempt from state laws that prohibit discrimination against certain classes of providers and consumer groups. They may legally be allowed to refer only to physicians and not include psychologists in their plans. Usually, only minimal levels of mental health coverage are included, and they often fail to meet the needs of certain patients, including children with special needs.

The variations on PPOs are limited:

1   Standard PPO plans include: (a) select provider panels, (b) negotiated payment rates for preferred providers, (c) rapid payment terms, (d) utilization management, and (e) consumer choice.

2   Exclusive provider organizations (EPOs) are like PPOs in their organization and purpose, but are more like HMOs in practical terms, as they require enrollees to use their contracted providers. They may or may not require a "gatekeeper" to access services.

Major Medical/Indemnity Insurance

This category was the most common type of insurance available before the development of HMOs and PPOs. Major medical insurance generally is designed to provide protection for above-average medical expenses, such as those that result from hospitalization or chronic illness. Consumers generally have a choice of deductible levels as well as the broadest choice of health care providers and facilities. Providers may agree to accept the assignment of insurance benefits and file claims for the consumer or may ask for payment at the time of service and require the consumer to file his or her own insurance claims.

Major medical plans, HMOs, and PPOs are usually regulated differently by state insurance codes because their financial structures are very different. There is a "safety net" for insurance companies, including PPOs, that protects the consumer and provider against bankruptcy. However, there generally is no safety net for HMOs (they are required to provide their own safety nets), so if the HMO goes bankrupt, the *provider* is at risk for the financial liability. A *capitated provider* is at the greatest risk, financially. That is, if a clinician agrees to join a capitated plan, he or she receives a set total payment, regardless of the actual services provided (this is discussed further in later sections).

Employee Assistance Plans

While not health insurance per se, employee assistance programs (EAPs) are often offered by large employers to provide targeted, short-term interventions to their employees without the cost of going to a psychologist or other mental health provider. Since EAPs generally do not provide services to children, they will not be reviewed here. Interested clinicians may wish to read the *EAP Digest* for updates on EAP practice. This magazine, published by Performance Resource Press, can be ordered by calling 1-800-453-7733. Winegar (1996) also provides a more comprehensive review.

MANAGED BEHAVIORAL HEALTH CARE

Managed behavioral health care (or mental health services) is usually provided as a "carve-out" benefit from a more comprehensive benefit package. Carve-out refers to a situation where an employer contracts with one health care company to manage medical coverage and with a different company specializing in managing mental health and substance abuse services (a managed behavioral health care company). The identity of the third-party payor or managed care company determines which laws and regulations apply to it. Managed behavioral health care organizations (MBHOs) that have contracted with federal or state governments to provide services (such as Medicaid, Medicare, or CHAMPUS) must comply with the federal and/or state laws and regulations governing provider contracting, incentive programs, and fraud and abuse. If the plan is employer sponsored (self-funded), it may be subject to provisions of the Employee Retirement Income Security Act, also known as ERISA, which preempt certain state laws. MBHOs are usually not *directly* regulated by the states, only as they fit within a law or regulation designed for another type of health provider or insurance entity. In contracting to provide services, clinicians should keep in mind that when an entity arranges for the delivery of health care services and assumes some or all of the financial risk for the cost of that care, it may be conducting a health insurance business or acting as an HMO, both of which usually require licensure by the state. MBHOs that operate under capitated arrangements are like insurers because they assume a degree of financial risk. They are unlike typical HMOs because they offer only one service. Some states allow these MBHO capitated entities to be licensed as a particular type of insurer, with requirements similar to HMOs. Therefore, before becoming party to a MBHO, the clinician should assure himself or herself that the entity is properly licensed for that type of business (Pollard & Tilson, 1996).

WATCHING MANAGED CARE COMPANIES

National Committee for Quality Assurance (NCQA)

The National Committee for Quality Assurance (NCQA) is a nonprofit organization whose stated purpose is to evaluate and report on the quality of managed care plans. The NCQA is composed of representatives from health plans, labor organizations, consumer groups, quality assurance experts, regulators, employers, and medicine. The NCQA is funded by volunatry fees from HMO and managed care reviews. Miller (1996a) criticized the NCQA's self-description as a "watchdog" over the managed care industry, stating "the managed care industry is the master of the NCQA *watchdog*, and this dog is guarding the industry's profits from the proponents of true accountability and effective regulation. The NCQA appears to be structured as an independent nonprofit organization [but] . . . it is an extension of the HMO industry" (p. 133). Since all of the NCQA's funds come from HMOs, promoting HMOs and other managed care entities actually benefits NCQA directly, such that criticizing, and therefore potentially harming, the managed care industry would decrease its funding sources.

The Behavioral Healthcare Task Force is the group that established accreditation standards for mental health or "behavioral health" managed care plans. This group is composed of representatives of the managed care industry with a few invited others. The Practice Directorate of the APA provided feedback on the initial proposed guidelines and raised four substantial objections to the draft standards:

1	Confidentiality is not adequately protected because managed behavioral health care organizations are allowed too much access to patient files.
2	Access to appropriate and timely care, with an appropriate and qualified provider, is not ensured by these standards.
3	There is an overreliance on psychiatrists and failure to recognize the qualifications of doctorally trained psychologists to perform certain duties.
4	When treatment is denied or providers are not credentialed, there is inadequate due process allowed (Vein & Cullen, 1996).

Miller (1996a) has delineated several other problems with the NCQA standards. He states, "These Standards do not set clear observable criteria, do not publicly report the information necessary for comparing the performance of one company to another, and do not give meaningful protection to the consumer" (p. 134). It remains to be seen how much influence organizations like the APA will have on the NCQA and other industry groups in their efforts to improve quality of mental health services accessed through a managed care system.

Health Plan Employer Data and Information Set

Health Plan Employer Data and Information Set (HEDIS) is a set of performance standards developed and used by the NCQA to rate managed care plans. The current version, HEDIS 3.0, was implemented in 1997 and includes revisions to the previous system. The new version requires more outcome measures (including a uniform customer satisfaction measure), includes Medicare and Medicaid recipients, and includes "test" items being evaluated for future use. However, mental health is not specifically included in HEDIS 3.0.

The Legal Center for Patient Protection

A nonprofit organization was formed in March 1997 to use litigation as the means to eliminate managed care abuses. Established by psychologists and psychiatrists with attorney litigators, the Legal Center for Patient Protection seeks to file lawsuits against major managed care companies on behalf of providers and

patients. The center believes that suits will make the companies more accountable for abuses and exploitation of patient care by impacting them financially
(on the "bottom line," the most important aspect of a managed care company's
existence). Suits have been filed and publicity received about denial of benefits
and poor services for serious mental health problems under managed care
coverage. Clinicians may contribute to the Legal Center to sustain its activities
and receive a newsletter (The Legal Center for Patient Protection, 1155 Con-
necticut Avenue NW, Suite 300, Washington, DC 20036. Phone: 202-429-6530;
fax: 202-332-8710).

National Coalition of Mental Health Professionals and Consumers, Inc

As a result of consumers' and professionals' dissatisfaction with managed care,
a grassroots organization, The National Coalition of Mental Health Professionals
and Consumers, Inc, was formed to inform the public of the negative impact of
managed mental health care (for information, call 516-424-5242 or access the
World Wide Web: http://www.cmhc.com/). This and other advocacy groups,
along with professional organizations such as the APA (and coalitions of other
organizations with which it affiliates), have helped spur the increasing number
of state and federal laws passed to protect consumers from inappropriate limits
on services (see Chapter 3) and providers from restrictions limiting their ability
to serve their patients' needs.

CONCLUSIONS

Each of the vignettes opening this chapter demonstrates some aspect of the ways
clinicians can respond to the managed care revolution. Not all of the suggestions
and responses will work for everyone, but clinicians *can* manage their practices
within and outside of managed care. Further changes in health care financing
will take place over the next several years. These changes will include minor
tinkering and eliminating some gross and easily publicized failures such as
"drive-through childbirth" and outpatient mastectomies (Church, 1997). More
dramatic changes will also occur when consumers of mental health services
recognize they have been shortchanged by the financing systems and demand
greater access and higher quality care than has been promulgated under the
current structures (Sleek, 1997). In addition, changes in state and federal law
will help curtail the abuses of managed care across a broad spectrum.

Problems Posed by Managed Care for Services to Children and Families

A 6-year-old girl was previously seen for six sessions by a child psychologist for behavior problems, anger, anxiety, and similar problems. The parents requested additional visits after the child revealed traumatic sexual abuse by the stepfather. The psychologist agreed that therapy was needed and contacted the HMO to request additional visits. The request was denied because there was no specific "problem" that could be resolved within a few sessions. The psychologist appealed the denial and was eventually granted several therapy sessions.

A psychologist on an inpatient psychiatric unit requested inpatient hospitalization for a 9-year-old boy who had twice tried to jump in front a moving vehicle. The managed care company would only certify the child for partial hospitalization rather than the requested inpatient care. The psychologist felt there was a real need for inpatient care because of the risk of the child making another suicide attempt, and felt an ethical obligation to inform the parents of this. She told the family what their insurance company had approved, and also stated what she recommended. The family complained to the managed care company, which told the psychologist not to voice to the family any disagreements with the company. The psychologist believed she had done the right thing, but became concerned that her service would be dropped from the managed care panel.

A family began seeing a psychologist for treatment of their child's problem. After four sessions, the family agreed that it was quite helpful and they wished to continue. Up to this point, they had paid for services out-of-pocket, but since this was likely to continue for several more sessions, they decided to go ahead and use their managed care benefits. However, when the psychologist requested approval for additional sessions, the request was denied due to a preexisting condition. The managed care organization stated that because the family had already seen the psychologist for this problem, the condition was pre-existing and the managed care plan did not have to pay for any further sessions.

In this chapter, we review the problems inherent in a system where cost-containment is the primary driving force, and the problems experienced by children and their families in accessing services in a managed care system, including restrictions imposed by utilization review, "medical necessity" restrictions, and limited access to specialists. In addition, we will review problems experienced by clinicians attempting to join managed care panels.

NEED FOR CHILD AND FAMILY SERVICES

Almost 30 years ago, the Joint Commission on the Mental Health of Children concluded that the status of mental health services for children was clearly inadequate (Friedman & Kutash, 1992). We do not believe this situation has been improved with the advent of managed care. In fact, it is likely that managed care's inherent economics cause it to lower mental health services to an insufficient level for effective treatment (Miller, 1996b). It is estimated that over 20% of all youth have a diagnosable mental disorder at any one point in time, and both the severity and prevalence of these problems are increasing. A 1989 survey found that among U.S. children ages 3–5, 9.5% had an emotional, developmental, or learning problem. Among 12- to 17-year-olds, the estimate was 25%. Among groups such as foster children, the incidence of mental and learning disorders is significantly higher than in the general population: More than 70% of foster children were diagnosed with Serious Emotional Disorders and were in need of mental health services according to the same study (Takayama, Bergman, & Connell, 1994).

The onset of mental disorders is occurring earlier, with such serious diagnoses as major depression recognized in preschoolers. The average age of onset of alcoholism has changed from the late 20s to the early 20s or late teens. All of these problems of children are compounded by changes in familial, social, and cultural supports for children. Reported cases of child maltreatment doubled from 1974 to 1980, and they quadrupled from 1974 to 1989. More and more children live in poverty with its attendant stresses (Friedman & Kutash, 1992).

Mental health services currently are fragmented and uncoordinated, resulting in inaccessible, limited, or overlapping services and wasted funds. Prevention services are often not reimbursed, despite evidence that these services can be cost-effective.

Over 14 million children are currently in need of outpatient mental health care, yet less than 2% of all adolescents in the United States accessed any type of mental health services in 1986, significantly less than the estimated incidence of problems in this population. During the 1970s and 1980s, with the increase of community-based care centers, it was expected that child utilization of public psychiatric inpatient hospitals would significantly decrease. However, only modest decreases were actually observed in inpatient utilization rates. These decreases were more than offset by large increases in admissions to private psychiatric hospitals because these services were covered by insurance policies, while outpatient services were not. Episodes of residential and inpatient care for children increased by 87% between 1980 and 1985. A 1990 study of private health insurance found that inpatient adolescent treatment expenses increased by 65% between 1986 and 1988. Many of those hospitalized could have been treated more appropriately and less expensively on an outpatient basis if the health insurance reimbursement structure had allowed it. Few data are available on outpatient utilization in the 1980s, and even less is available on private practice utilization. However, estimates of utilization vary from 1–3% for ambulatory mental health care for adolescents during the 1980s (Padgett, Patrick, Burns, Schlesinger, & Cohen, 1993).

The public strongly supports adequate care for children. A 1993 opinion poll found that 73% of Americans stated that children's health and education was their number one priority for the new Clinton Administration (APA Practice Directorate, 1996). Most Americans agreed that children and their families need access to high-quality mental health care that includes prevention and early intervention as well as crisis management.

Managed care was created as a result of escalating health care costs. It was assumed that a majority of the skyrocketing costs was due to the economic incentives of traditional indemnity insurance, which often reimbursed insured enrollees for 80% of their medical expenses after their deductible was met. Unfortunately, in many ways, the managed care movement has not met the high goals of providing accessible, affordable, and appropriate care. As a primary impact, managed care has served to decrease outpatient mental health services even though outpatient treatment already had built-in cost controls in place (through copayments and deductibles) and outpatient treatment is the less expensive alternative to costly inpatient care. In addition, the costs of administering a managed care plan use up many of the limited dollars available for mental health treatment. All of this results in fewer patients served, often with those receiving services being undertreated (Miller, 1996b).

ACCESSIBILITY OF SERVICES

Availability of mental health benefits and services affects utilization by children. Children with little or no mental health insurance use mental health services far less than those who have mental health insurance. The type of benefit plan available also affects utilization. In one study, those enrolled in a "high option" plan (20% copay, $100 deductible, no caps), with more covered benefits, accessed more services (Padgett et al., 1993). The high option users averaged 4.6 more visits than low option enrollees in 1978 and 4.9 more visits in 1983. Thus, this study found that the benefit plan had a clear and dramatic effect both on the likelihood a child would enter outpatient mental health treatment and on the number of visits. The insurance available, not the need for treatment, determined the length of treatment for children. Children enrolled in high option plans were almost three times as likely to use mental health services as those in low option plans. Children who may have needed treatment may not have received it because of lack of insurance.

One of the problems of accessing services has to do with reducing what are considered extraneous services versus reducing clearly needed services. As has been stated, children's mental health needs are still largely unmet in the United States. Therefore, cost savings achieved through denial of services results in even more children being untreated or undertreated. The ramifications of inadequate access to child and family services are serious. Not only will children experience distress in childhood, but as they mature into adulthood their problems may exacerbate. The concepts of early intervention, prevention of problems, and promotion of mental health were goals in the early generations of HMOs (and remain in the advertising literature from managed care organizations). In reality, these ideals are largely dropped because of the need for managed care companies to demonstrate short-term profits. Although the need and the logic exist for providing appropriate mental health care for children and adolescents, managed care achieves cost savings through denial of services.

COST CONTAINMENT AND UTILIZATION

The intent of managed care was to save money by improving efficiencies, reducing redundant and unnecessary services ("waste"), and coordinating necessary services. However, over time, it has become apparent that such cost-containment strategies have been inadequate to maintain the profit needed. The current basis of managed care focuses on capitation, or limits placed on the total number of dollars available, so the total cost of all services to all enrollees of the plan must be kept within budget (i.e., below the actual costs in order to turn a profit for the company's shareholders). The reimbursement limit is often set relatively low for this reason, with incentives established to stay well within the limits (e.g., those who help save the company money get to share in that money). There is, by design, an orientation to save money by restricting or not providing services in a variety of ways in addition to paying considerably lower fees to health care providers. Managed care companies claim the cost savings come from greater efficiencies and reduction of "unnecessary" services through these procedures.

QUALITY OF CARE ISSUES

While managed care arrangements appear to produce an initial cost savings that does not continue over the long term, Miller (1996b) asserts that managed care has been harmful to outpatient mental health services because the more intense focus on cost savings has forced these organizations to abandon any commitment to quality care. To save money, essential services are cut or limited. Psychologists from across the country have reported problems with undertreatment in the managed care system, sometimes resulting in adverse consequences and often resulting in slower progress in therapy (APA Practice Directorate, 1996). In several surveys, psychologists strongly report that managed care negatively affects the quality of treatment (Bowers & Knapp, 1993; Sinnett & Holen, 1993; Widmeyer Group, Inc., 1994). In studies with adult patients, Miller and Luft (1994) found that fewer depressed patients were properly diagnosed under managed care than under fee-for-service plans and that primary care physicians (the managed care organization's gatekeeper) failed to correctly identify depression more than half the time. In addition, depressed patients who received treatment under a managed care plan had worse outcomes, in some cases even deteriorating, than those treated in a fee-for-service setting. Almost every child clinician practicing within a managed care system of some sort likely has one or more stories of an intrusive and incorrect assessment or treatment decision forced on the clinician by a managed care gatekeeper. For example, a report on a very early prepaid system noted that an adolescent girl diagnosed with anorexia nervosa was treated through intermittent interventions rather than in continuous comprehensive care (Bennett & Gavalya, 1982). The clinical vignettes presented in this book represent other such situations.

A second problem of quality of care is seen in the trend to reduce the number of visits for psychotherapy to very low levels, often only three or four sessions. In 1989, 95% of insurance policies had limits on outpatient mental health benefits (Miller, 1996b). Research shows that type and availability of insurance affects the amount of therapy received, but there is little research supporting any "ultrabrief" therapy. In fact, only those patients with very mild concerns, which are often not covered by managed care insurance at all, consistently show improvements with very short treatments of three or four sessions; those with more severe problems require more intense and/or longer treatment (Miller, 1996b). The literature on brief therapy traditionally defines it as 15–30 sessions. Additionally, many of the treatment protocols described for children's problems require 12 sessions or longer to complete. These interventions would be considered long-term therapy under most managed care plans, rather than being typical for brief therapy. Patients requiring such "long-term" therapy are often expected to be referred to cheaper interventions such as medication management, self-help groups, or other sources of help outside the managed care plan, even before their maximum allowable number of visits has been used.

Other unpublished reports of underdiagnosis of psychological problems by gatekeeper physicians, failure to make appropriate referrals, and inadequate follow-up circulate among clinicians. Many conclude that, as provider fees are squeezed and paperwork and telephone conference demands increase, managed care has taken dollars that could have been used for patient care and used them for administrative expenses or to return profits to shareholders and large salaries to management. Audits have found that little of the premium paid goes directly to patient care and that utilization data are often grossly overreported.

ADMINISTRATIVE COSTS OF MANAGED CARE

To illustrate the extreme cost of managed care, Miller (1996b) stated that administrative expenses and profit in a managed care company can run from 25–65% of the funds available, whereas under traditional indemnity insurance, only about 2% of the funds available for mental health care are used for administrative expenses. Administrative costs are always difficult to estimate (especially from outside an organization), although it is clear that running a managed care company takes dollars away from patient care. As managed care plans evolve, there are not enough funds available to pay for administrative expenses or to reduce the copayment requirements and still achieve cost savings unless services are also drastically reduced.

ACCESSING SERVICES WITHIN A MANAGED CARE ENVIRONMENT

Accessibility of psychological services for patients is a major problem because managed care organizations achieve cost savings through restricting access to providers. Restrictions on services may be made by limiting the number of providers on a panel, making it difficult to get appointments or physically get to the provider, by delaying the referral to a provider, or by diagnosing the patient's problems via a telephone interview and referring to the cheapest form of care. Patients rarely know the details of any cost-control mechanisms that may affect a managed care company's decisions to refer to specialists or to recommend specific treatment options. For example, many managed care organizations require that patients with certain diagnoses be referred to a psychiatrist for medication management (Browning & Browning, 1996), even when the patient is a child and the parents do not wish to have their child placed on medication. When such referrals are not followed-up on or are refused, the gatekeeper/reviewer at the managed care company may deny all further requests for treatment because the patient refused to accept the reviewer's recommendation. Even providers who have signed legal contracts are often unaware of the workings of the managed care system with which they have contracted.

Although mental health services for children may be available through the schools and other settings (e.g., pediatric hospitals), more mental health service providers are needed to address the vast array of problems children and families currently face. The services available through these settings are often difficult for families to access because they are usually underfunded, maximally utilized, and often inadequate to serve the number and variety of problems presented. At present, mental health services for children and their families are often inaccessible, limited, fragmented, or overlapping.

Even though targeted at the same problems of children, funds from various sources (health, mental health, special education, juvenile justice, and child welfare) are often inflexible and uncoordinated. Indirect or preventive activities (school consultation, primary care consultation, case management) are often not reimbursable, despite the fact that these services are cost-effective. When services are reimbursable, such as through Medicaid, they are often bogged down in paperwork demands and bureaucracy. In cases such as child maltreatment, prevention is clearly preferable to remedial treatment, yet these services are not usually covered by health insurance plans. For example, parent training and in-home family supportive therapy that strengthens the family before any abuse occurs are far better than the need for child protection services, foster care, legal involvement, and the disruption of family lives (APA Practice Directorate, 1996).

Accessing adequate mental health services for children, adolescents, and families was notably difficult even before the latest generation of managed care arrangements (e.g., Knitzer, 1982, 1993; Saxe, Cross, & Silverman, 1988). Under these new circumstances, children and their parents are likely to be even further restricted in accessing appropriate care.

Other factors that influence utilization of mental health services are availability of providers, parental income, and ethnicity, with higher-income earners and whites accessing more services than others and those in cities with more providers accessing services more frequently. As benefit plans change, more children are receiving some mental health services, but their amount of use is decreasing, largely due to changes in insurance. Cost-sharing and caps on treatment appear to affect length of treatment, whether or not more or longer treatment is needed (Padgett et al., 1993). Mental health services should promote psychological competence and self-sufficiency rather than focus exclusively on dysfunction and pathology. This is especially true for children, for whom prevention and early intervention can have long-lasting benefits to the child, the family, and society.

Outpatient treatment is clearly less expensive than inpatient treatment. However, managed care attempts to limit the use of such outpatient treatment. This might be a reasonable thing to do if outpatient mental health treatment were being overused, but research studies clearly indicate that it is not. Indeed, far fewer children and adolescents actually access mental health services than are in need of such services. Moreover, outpatient mental health treatment has generally been limited by high copayments and deductibles in indemnity-type insurance plans. High out-of-pocket expenses have made consumers cost-conscious about their spending for mental health services. Consumers self-paid between 45% and 48% of the money spent on psychotherapy as indicated in a 1987 survey (Miller, 1996b). In 1988, 76% of insurance policies had copayment requirements of 50% or greater, and 77% of policies had payment limits of $1000 or less. From a managed care perspective, copayments are attractive ways to limit costs because insurance policies with 50% copayments have been shown to lower the cost of mental health services as much as 60% below those policies with no copayments, primarily by decreasing the number of patients served. Therefore, as managed care attempts to further reduce utilization of mental health services, there is a very real risk of cutting services below what is psychologically necessary for many individuals.

When unrealistic limits are placed on the number of visits allowed or by having very low caps on dollars spent, the quality and appropriateness of mental health care is often inadequate (Higuchi, 1994). Although more individuals may be seen under these plans, they are often seen only long enough to identify a problem but not long enough to provide adequate, if any, treatment. For example, if the maximum cap on mental health services is $500 for a patient, the entire year's benefit can be used before a complete assessment (parent interview, child interview, psychometric testing) is done. Although the mental health parity law effective in 1998 removes this barrier in a few cases, in most cases it (or similar barriers) will remain. As a result, it is likely that an increasing portion of the population is denied access to needed mental health services, those receiving services are underserved, and those with moderate to severe problems are being denied services beyond brief, crisis-oriented help (Miller, 1996b). Mental health services are already being provided in the schools and in primary care settings, but much more is needed in order to address the extensive array of problems faced by children and families.

CURRENT PROCEDURAL TERMINOLOGY CODES

Many managed care companies require billing using Current Procedural Terminology, or CPT, Codes (American Medical Association, 1996), which are standard procedure codes used to identify services provided by physicians and other health care providers. Psychiatric and mental health procedures are generally billed under 908XX codes, although at times, neurology and other code groups have been used. Recently, psychological testing has been changed to a 96100 code, and it is anticipated that other codes may change in the future. In general, managed care companies tie reimbursement to procedures for one's licensure. In other words, even though a neuropsychologist might appropriately bill under neurology procedure codes, because the provider is a psychologist, the managed care company may only pay for mental health codes. This varies from company to company, so the clinician must check on any particular managed care organization's policies.

The most common codes used by the child clinician include the following:

- 90801—intake diagnostic interview (generally only one or two visits per child per episode are allowed)
- 90830 (96100 as of 1996, but some companies still use older codes)—psychological testing per hour (authorized in either a preset number of hours regardless of problem or in an individually determined number of hours based on the clinician's request and reviewed by the managed care organization's representative)
- 90843—20- to 30-minute individual therapy session
- 90844—45- to 50-minute individual therapy session
- 90847—family therapy (often not covered by managed care)
- 90853—group therapy (not covered by some managed care organizations)

Inpatient and outpatient codes are generally the same, although inpatient procedures may be billed by a different provider, and there may be limits on who or how many providers can bill during an inpatient cycle. It is wise for the clinician to clarify these issues prior to providing services in either an inpatient or outpatient setting.

REDUCED FEES FOR CLINICIAN-PROVIDERS

One primary method of reducing the costs to the managed care company providing mental health services is by reducing the fees paid to the providers. That is, when a clinician signs the contract to join a managed care provider panel, he or she agrees to accept the fee schedule determined by the company. These fees are often well below what the clinician might normally charge and collect.

The January 1995 Survey Report from *Psychotherapy Finances* indicated that psychologists' average fees (usual and customary for fee-for-service patients per session) was $90 ("Fee," 1995). This average fee represented 82% of the psychiatrists' average fee for the same service. When a managed care organization was the payor, the average fee was $75 per session for psychologists (and roughly the same difference from psychiatrists' fees). However, when other third parties paid (such as major medical insurance), the fee reimbursement was the same as what was collected from private pay patients: $90. In general, psychologists' fees were $15–$20 higher than other, nonpsychiatrist mental health providers (social workers, counselors, marriage and family therapists). It should be noted that in this survey, respondents indicated they were receiving two-thirds of their income from non-managed care sources. Therefore, the group may not be representative of some markets or practice conditions. In fact, the Survey Report stated that the results do not "reflect the experiences of those who have fallen by the wayside; abandoning therapy practice, taking salaried jobs, or just feeling too discouraged to fill out the questionnaire" (p. 1). More recently, *Psychotherapy Finances* (1996) reported that rates for group therapy varied from $20–$60 per 1½ hour session and that managed care rates were generally $25–$45 for group therapy ("Therapy Groups," 1996).

Managed care "discounts" tend to vary from 0% (payment of the provider's regular full fee) to more than 50% in noncapitated plans. The financial health of the managed care organization appears to be a significant factor in setting fees, as does the level of development (or "generation") of the managed care entity (Miller, 1996b). Miller notes that "first-generation" managed care organizations tend to discount fees less and to collect higher copayments. As the managed care entity evolves, fees are reduced and providers bear increasingly greater risk until ultimately the plan becomes capitated, with providers accepting the majority of the risk and accepting significantly reduced fees if they continue to provide the services. This issue is further discussed in Chapter 5.

Because of reduced fees the clinician will have difficulty maintaining the level of income at the same rate of workload. This problem is further compounded by the "withholds" that are usually kept out of fee payments to the clinician. These are usually outlined in the provider contract, and the amount of money withheld is presumably given to the provider at the end of the contract year when the health plan budget balances out. No interest payments are added to the withhold and there is always a distinct possibility that no payment will be forthcoming should the plan run in the red for the year. Sometimes the fees are withheld even without the provider's agreement (e.g., Cantor, 1997).

GATEKEEPERS

Access to managed care services, other than primary care, is most often through a "gatekeeper," which could be the patient's primary care physician (PCP) or an employee of the managed care company. A "gatekeeper" determines who gets services, from whom, and for how long. The gatekeeper is sometimes a PCP, often with financial incentives to minimize use of a system's services. Increasingly, clinicians are finding nonclinician gatekeepers with credentials that are neither relevant nor useful to their job demands (e.g., HMO staff employees with a variety of college degrees, reading from a protocol handbook, but who still must attempt to minimize system utilization). The lowest level of gatekeeper does not usually have to be a "like provider" (i.e., with training in the same field of expertise as the provider) and may have little or no training in mental health. Patients are often not informed about the financial incentives offered to both the PCP and the company employee for limiting referrals to psychologists and other specialists. Indeed, the advertising copy often describes the first contact as helping the patient find the services he or she needs. Of course, the managed care company has a financial stake in defining what that "need" is and how it will be handled. The managed care organizations would rarely call their case managers (representatives) or PCP a gatekeeper because the implication is that a gatekeeper is keeping the gates closed as opposed to being a gate-opener or care facilitator.

There are no definitive, impartial studies proving either that gatekeepers reduce costs, or that they do not: There are studies that show both outcomes. Gatekeepers do add to the costs of administering services. However, under the gatekeeper model, more generally trained providers are expected to provide more and more specialty care, for which they are often unprepared and which care they may not provide appropriately. We believe that the more care placed in the hands of less-qualified providers (either because of lack of specialization or lack of advanced training), the lower the quality of those services will be. The less qualified provider may underdiagnose, misrefer, or maltreat significant problems.

UTILIZATION MANAGEMENT/UTILIZATION REVIEW

Following the initial visit, in most cases, the clinician on a managed care panel is generally responsible for contacting the managed care company for authorization for any additional visits or for testing. This contact occurs through a telephone call to the gatekeeper or, more often, through paper forms. UR is the process whereby the managed care company determines whether the requested services are "medically necessary," and therefore covered, services under the patient's insurance plan. The stated purpose of UR is to improve cost-effectiveness while maintaining quality of care and to decrease abuse of services.

UR developed out of a belief that the dramatic increase in health care spending was because of unnecessary or poor-quality care. Consequently, requiring review and approval in advance was originally intended to improve the quality and efficiency of health care. It has, unfortunately, evolved into simply a means of saving money. Originally intended for inpatient services, it has been applied increasingly to outpatient care. Indeed, there is more and more pressure to increase UR for outpatient mental health services. The utilization reviewers' jobs depend on saving their employers' money. This self-interest may mean that they cannot be totally objective in reviewing treatment requests. (Admittedly, providers' requests for more sessions are not isolated from their own financial self-interests either.) Companies providing UR procedures have to limit expenditures for patient treatment in order to pay for their own costly review services (Miller, 1996b). There are few data demonstrating that UR actually saves money. If it does, the savings are usually small. In addition, studies suggest that as cost-savings mechanisms become more effective nationally, quality declines (Zusman, 1990).

Features of UR Statutes

Most states have utilization review statutes on the books that regulate aspects of UR, including those performed by managed care companies and insurance carriers. It is important for clinicians to become familiar with their state's UR statutes and, specifically, to be familiar with the following features:

- The definition of "health care provider," and whether this includes psychologists; this definition will determine who is considered qualified to conduct reviews at various stages
- Whether there is a "like provider" requirement, which states that a reviewer must be licensed and competent to perform the same services as the ones he or she is reviewing
- Confidentiality provisions pertaining to patient records, and any restrictions on conducting telephone reviews
- Grievance and appeals procedures
- Prohibitions against monetary incentives that are tied to the reviewer's decision

■ Whether managed care companies are required to disclose their UR decision-making criteria and provide summaries to clinicians (providers) and patients

Managed care companies which are not required by law to disclose information regarding procedures and criteria for conducting reviews are sometimes reluctant to do so. However, clinicians should request the information as a matter of course.

Clinician's Involvement in UR

UR involves substantial costs to the clinician in terms of time spent making telephone calls, in case reviews, and completing paperwork. Those costs to the clinician are not reimbursed, but must be absorbed, resulting in decreased income and availability (Borenstein, 1990; Zusman, 1990). The core functions of UR include eligibility determination, benefit interpretation, and precertification for inpatient admission or outpatient services. Eligibility determination verifies that the patient is actually a member of the insurance plan and is eligible to receive the services requested. It can be either the patient's or clinician's responsibility to make the initial contact with the insurance plan. Even if it is designated as the patient's responsibility, it is often wise for the clinician to verify coverage independently on or close to the date of service, as people often change jobs or have other changes in eligibility that may not have been noted previously and that may affect their eligibility for benefits. In doing so, the clinician may avoid providing a service that is ultimately denied reimbursement, unless other arrangements are made.

The clinician participates in interpretation of benefits by assessing the patient and providing a diagnosis. If the diagnosis is a covered one (i.e., defined as "medically necessary"), benefits may be approved (the clinician may provide the prescribed services with a good chance of being reimbursed). If it is not, benefits may be denied. For example, many patients present with "V-Code" diagnoses, such as v61.20—Parent-Child Relational Problem, which are not covered in many benefit packages. The clinician then faces an ethical dilemma: Does the child actually meet the criteria for another diagnosis that is covered by the plan, such as Oppositional Defiant Disorder or Adjustment Disorder with Disturbance of Conduct? If not, the proposed therapy may not be a covered benefit, and the patient and her family may go away disappointed and distressed that they could not get help for their real problem. The clinician has then lost a potential patient and the income from that therapy, and the patient has lost the opportunity to make changes that would improve presenting functioning and may prevent the occurrence of a more serious problem in the future. We think it is likely that some children are given more serious diagnoses in order for treatment of the problems to be covered under managed care plans. If a clinician is unsure whether a particular diagnosis or treatment is covered, he or she can call the managed care plan reviewer and ask. If it is not, the clinician has other options, such as making a referral to an agency with a sliding scale or no-fee arrangement, or informing the family that the diagnosis is not covered by their benefit plan but that therapy is available on a fee-for-service basis with the clinician. However, families are less likely to use services that are not covered by their insurance.

TREATMENT PROTOCOLS

Most mental health benefit plans set access and treatment rules or protocols applicable only to adult patients. These rules are referred to by various terms, such as treatment algorithms, practice guidelines, standards of care, clinical pathways, and managed care paths or tracks, with some variations in the accepted treatment procedures and how rigidly they are applied. (Many of the protocols used by managed care are considered proprietary information in that they cannot be publicly displayed.) Few companies have separate UR procedures or templates for children, and almost none have guidelines for children with special needs. Some plans do not cover partial hospitalization programs or residential treatment programs, and few cover community-based interventions, such as school visits and classroom management plans. Where guidelines for children do exist, they are often overly restrictive or inappropriate. We know of more than one plan where assessment of a child to obtain a diagnosis of ADHD by a psychologist is not a covered benefit, although the medication for treating ADHD is covered. In another plan, Ritalin (methylphenidate) is not covered (not included in the plan's approved drug formulary), but other medications for ADHD are allowed.

PRECERTIFICATION

Precertification decisions are made by employees of the managed care plan, before an individual enters into outpatient therapy or is admitted to an inpatient unit. Utilization reviewers are generally available 24 hours a day to make such determinations. The purpose of precertification is to save costs by allowing the least costly care that is deemed appropriate (e.g., partial hospitalization versus inpatient treatment; intensive outpatient therapy versus residential treatment). Managed care plans vary in their demands for precertification, with some companies allowing a fairly large number of visits without review and others requiring each visit to be individually approved. Obviously, the more review required, the greater the cost to both the managed care plan and the clinician. This extended and repeated review process can be quite disruptive to therapy if patients need to wait 10–14 days between visits to allow for this approval of visits. On the other hand, managed behavioral health care plans that authorize up to 12 visits without any additional review can expedite delivery of services in a more cost-effective manner. That is, most patients complete therapy within 12 visits or less, with the majority (75%) completing in 10–12 visits, so the expense of a review is avoided.

When a limited number of visits is authorized initially and additional treatment is needed, it is necessary for the clinician to justify to the managed care reviewer the need for these services. To do so effectively, it is critical to keep thorough enough chart notes to be able to tell what has been done, what has been accomplished, and what the plan is for the next several visits, in terms of objective goals for outcome. If the clinician is unsure of what type of goals are generally approved by the reviewers for a plan, it is permissible to ask the reviewer for examples of some well-written (in their opinion) goals. The clinician can then use these as templates for writing future goals for that company. If the plan relies on diagnosis-related groups (DRGs), the clinician should ask what the typical and preferred types and durations of treatment are for the diagnoses in which he or she is most interested.

CONCURRENT REVIEW

Concurrent review is another type of treatment authorization, but it occurs during the course of treatment rather than prior to treatment. There is some amount of risk to the provider that the reviewer will not authorize services that have already been accessed. In this case, the patient is generally responsible for the costs of unauthorized treatment. Patients are often reluctant to access services prior to knowing whether and at what level they will be covered.

DENIAL OF SERVICE AUTHORIZATION

If the clinician's request for authorization of services has been denied, he or she can and often should appeal. If a clinician believes that the treatment is needed and does not appeal its denial, the clinician may be held legally liable for any negative outcomes related to the withholding of that treatment (see Chapter 3). While the managed care company may share in this liability, the clinician will likely be in a better position to defend his or her actions if he or she has vigorously appealed the decision through all available channels. It is generally to the clinician's benefit to be thoroughly familiar with the appeals process for each managed care plan for which he or she is a provider. There is some risk in appealing decisions, as some managed care companies will terminate providers who appeal their decisions. The courts are currently examining this issue, and we hope there will soon be provisions in the law that prohibit this practice.

RESTRICTING PATIENTS' ACCESS TO SPECIALIST PROVIDERS

ERISA unintentionally reduced access to some mental health care and has allowed some self-insured benefit plans to exclude psychological services. ERISA-protected plans are exempt from state regulations that apply to other managed care companies. Therefore, some ERISA-protected plans legally exclude psychologists from being providers or require physicians to supervise psychologists, for example, which obviously restricts access to psychological services. These entities also tend to limit amounts of service or utilize only a limited number of psychologists, thus further limiting consumer access to their choice of providers and limiting access of psychologists to panels (Higuchi, 1994).

Managed care plans restrict the choices of referral sources, thus increasing potential problems caused by miscommunication with unfamiliar providers. Additionally, if a PCP gatekeeper is not familiar with a clinician's qualifications, he or she will be less confident in both the referral and the results. Some managed care companies may agree that visiting the specialist with the most knowledge initially is a better way to reduce costs than receiving several levels of ineffective care before seeing the appropriate specialist, but these companies are rare.

Many plans do not differentiate providers by age group served: Anyone willing to see a child for assessment or therapy may be listed and counted as a child psychologist, whether or not he or she has specific training to work with children. The clinician should inform referral sources of his or her unique qualifications and expertise, which can help increase the number of appropriate referrals received, while decreasing the number of inappropriate ones.

"MEDICAL NECESSITY" AND NONCOVERED DIAGNOSES

Several plans specifically exclude common childhood diagnoses, such as attention deficits and learning disorders, and some exclude all "child counseling." Even when diagnoses or treatments are covered, if a UR entity determines that the recommended care is not "medically necessary," coverage may be denied, although the patient's available benefits may not have been used up. When a clinician disagrees with a UR decision to deny services, he or she should respectfully but vigorously protest to the managed care company using the procedures outlined in the contract or agreements. If the clinician does not do this, he or she may be held legally liable for any negative outcomes resulting from those services being withheld.

Most managed care contracts provide reimbursement for only "medically necessary" services, but often fail to define a priori what is medically necessary. Managed care companies may attempt to impose restrictions and limits of care that are not disclosed in their benefit documents. Without reading the documents, the clinician would not be aware of the payor's different interpretation of what was offered to the patient-consumer. Clinicians can support their patients in asking for their rights by encouraging them to read their patient benefits publications and encouraging them to directly contact their employer's benefits office or the insurer to complain that they are not receiving what was promised. In addition, every practitioner should read and keep up-to-date on state laws and regulations affecting the provision of services in their state. States are becoming more and more active in requiring managed care companies to act responsibly and are protecting consumers and providers from abuses within the system. One possible remedy available to the patient is to complain to the state regulatory agency against their managed care company, stating that what they have advertised, either in public ads or in the patient's benefits handbook, is not what is being offered by the company ("bad faith claim"). This may or may not result in services being approved, and will likely take a very long time to accomplish. Meanwhile, the clinician must guard against unnecessary disruption in care.

WHAT DRIVES MANAGED CARE
(AND DRIVES PSYCHOLOGISTS ELSEWHERE)

Managed care is driven by a basic philosophy of cost savings. The promise to buyers is that the managed care organization will deliver a specific array of health care services at a cost that is lower than what would be paid on the open market. We have reviewed many of the ways managed care achieves these savings: limiting services, restricting access to services or to specialists, and contracting for reduced fees from providers, among others. To many clinicians, particularly psychologists, this approach to health care, specifically for mental health care, is contrary to their training and beliefs and produces some level of discomfort with the choices available. Does this mean ethical and competent clinicians cannot or should not work with managed care? No. Only that each individual must find the fit that is right for him or her.

There is a range of options available for clinicians working with managed care or avoiding managed care. On one extreme is the position espoused by Browning and Browning (1996) and Winegar and Bistline (1994) that clinicians should view employers or insurance companies as the true consumers of managed care therapy, with the benefits manager as the person who can best decide which services a patient should receive. Similarly, Austad and Hoyt (1992) suggest that clinicians within a managed care program must fit the treatment to the limits of the benefit package rather than determining the clinical or therapeutic needs of the patient and then helping him or her to access those services. This philosophy is contrary to what many psychologists believe to be ethical and competent practice because it places the interests of the employer or insurance company above those of the patient (Miller, 1996b).

On the other extreme, clinicians can choose to avoid managed care altogether. Such a decision in this day and age is likely to result in less income from private practice, and will probably require that the clinician pursue a variety of outside contracts or other sources of income. The threat of diminishing income is hard to accept for clinicians who have spent a number of years in graduate school in order to increase their skills and knowledge and, presumably, their incomes. There are a number of options between these two extremes, and each clinician will find his or her own comfort level somewhere along the line. In Chapter 5, we review some of the pros and cons of managed care; in Chapter 6, we outline how to practice outside the managed care system.

Legal and Ethical Issues for the Clinician in Managed Care

At the initial session with a patient and his parents, a clinician informed the parents about the limits on the number of psychotherapy sessions for the presenting problems given the family's membership in an HMO. This information, coupled with concerns over confidentiality of the information being sent to the managed care company, resulted in the parents deciding to pay "out of pocket" for the treatment.

A clinician, after completing paperwork for a claim for reimbursement for services to a child, received a denial of coverage for initial intake visits because the diagnosis section included "rule out ADHD." The company had determined that because ADHD was "incurable," no reimbursement was required. The clinician informed the patient's parent of this action. The parent consulted her benefits policy, which did not state any exclusionary clauses for certain diagnoses. She complained to her employer's benefits office and to the state insurance commissioner. The claim was eventually paid, but the clinician was dropped from the provider panel within 6 months.

The orientation of managed care and its general procedures pose challenges to the ethical and legal practice of psychology. In this chapter, we will outline some of the major issues with suggestions for resolving them. We will discuss some of the conflicts of interest that need to be resolved for ethical and legal practice in managing managed care. These issues include restriction of services, undertreatment, information disclosure, liability, appealing adverse coverage decisions, treatment beyond reimbursement, and confidentiality. Finally, we present an overview of managed care contract provisions.

Managed care plans differ regarding how the clinician will interact with the plans' managers about service coverage and authorization and payment for services. Some plans' clinicians are required to provide documents and information to the client, but not to file forms for reimbursement or to negotiate directly with the managed care gatekeepers. Other plans require clinicians to make direct contact and, correspondingly, to become advocates on behalf of the patient in dealing with the plan or network. Thus, these clinicians may spend several hours a week making telephone calls to gatekeepers and treatment reviewers. (Even if patients file the forms for their own reimbursement, having paid out of pocket for the clinician's charges, it will often be necessary for the clinician to interact with the managed care staff.) Managed care plans differ in their requirements for authorizing various out-of-network services. Some require extensive documents or information from out-of-network providers in order to authorize care, and some specify particular billing requirements, while others do not require any direct contact with non-network providers. For network providers, plans also vary in their requirements. Some require filing a brief form requesting several sessions of therapy, while others require weekly phone updates with a care manager. Some plans routinely approve up to a certain number of visits (say 8 or 10), while others allow only one or two visits per authorization. The administration and appeal time, which is always nonreimbursable, is a major complaint of many clinicians.

RESTRICTION OF SERVICES

There are conflicts of interest inherent in the managed care situation. As stated succinctly by Susan Wooley (1993): "Decisions about what is needed are made by members of a company whose profits depend on delivering as little service as possible" (p. 388). This inherent conflict leads directly to various methods of restricting services. The policy statement on managed care from the APA noted that "managed care delivery programs, by their very nature, frequently impose artificial and/or economic barriers to consumer access to health care services" (Fox, 1989, p. 1024). It is in the managed care company's profit interest not to provide services and then keep the money it would otherwise have to spend. Consequently, companies often impose restrictions on the types of problems covered, the types and range of services allowed, the eligibility for reimbursement, and the type or number of providers of the services. Typically, the more expensive services or most frequent problems will be restricted in order to reduce costs.

Limits on Diagnoses and Treatment

Policies and plans may differ even within the same locale. For example, in one area, we know that one plan will cover psychological treatment for ADHD for a certain number of sessions per year, but proper assessment procedures to secure a diagnosis are not reimbursed (one session for an interview is permitted); another plan will pay for full psychological assessment, but will not reimburse treatment for ADHD if diagnosed (because this condition is judged to be "incurable"). In other places, clinicians have been advised by clerks and fellow practitioners *not* to put "rule out ADHD" in their assessment/treatment plans because the managed care company clerks will automatically disallow coverage if ADHD is even suspected. This advice, however well-meaning, hinders the clinician in following his or her standard of practice and promotes subterfuge in dealing with managed care. Many times, however, the patient is not aware that the policy will exclude particular diagnoses or restrict certain services. For example, the plan's benefit brochure may describe 20 sessions of psychotherapy per year, but fail to note that there are restrictions on types of problems covered or that the therapy may be terminated in 5 or 6 sessions.

Limits on Benefits

Several plans offer such limits as a maximum of $500 per year in outpatient benefits, but allow only 50% of up to $50 per session or less (amounting to a $25 payment by the managed care entity!). Most psychologists in urban areas charge significantly more than $50 per session. The patient is obligated to pay the remainder out of pocket. Patient copayment generally results in decreased use of mental health benefits—and a cost saving for the patient's employer and the managed care company. However, this decreased use is not necessarily in the best interests of the patient. Furthermore, if the patient is not informed in advance of restrictions on services or cannot receive needed services, the presumed reason for having mental health benefits would be unattainable. Also, the clinician will suffer from a decreased income. Importantly, his or her ability to effect change with a patient may be impaired through inadequate time to work with a patient or family. Other managed care plans limit psychological testing to only 1 hour, but do not state this limitation in their patient benefits publications. Obviously this limited amount of time is quite restrictive and does not permit full and adequate assessment. Such restrictions are generally unanticipated by families seeking care. Families may hold the clinician responsible for not "getting my insurance company to pay for it." It is important that the clinician discuss insurance and benefits with patients at the first meeting and help them understand that the managed care entity is the one that sets the restrictions. The clinician can help them secure the benefits they are due, as best he or she can. If the clinician believes a test or treatment is necessary, the patient should be told what is necessary and why. The managed care company should not determine what the clinician believes is in the patient's best interest, only what it is willing to pay for.

While we strongly recommend that clinicians advise their patients to study their own benefit policies, some managed care contracts contain clauses binding the clinician to remain silent about restrictions that may appear to be criticism of the policies or the company. These "gag rules" are being removed, often after judicial rulings (and are discussed later in this chapter). Clinicians may mark out or delete parts of contracts they find objectionable, initialing all such changes. However, the legalities of such actions are not known, and the managed care plan may not allow such deletions. Discussion with the managed care company is probably the best action.

Our sense is that, despite managed care restrictions on services, most clinicians feel obligated to provide necessary services and procedures under their own professional standards, the prevailing local standards of care, and the discipline's ethical principles and practice guidelines.

Beliefs about Costs of Psychotherapy

Another potential problem with restricting services is that physicians, who are likely sources of the clinician's referrals, may believe that psychological services are more expensive than most families can afford and that treatment may last for months, thus making it prohibitively expensive. Because of these beliefs, in essence, they restrict services by not referring for psychological services. We suggest that, when talking with potential referral sources (physician, nurses, school personnel, and others), the clinician should give some idea of what a typical evaluation or treatment program for the identified problem might cost. As discussed in the section on developing a self-pay market, we suggest that the clinician not just provide a dollar figure for estimating usual costs of assessment and treatment, but also make comparisons to expenditures typically incurred for living expenses, such as the cost of painting a room, buying a set of tires, or buying a new television, while emphasizing the importance of psychological treatment (if justified). This information may overcome the parent's hesitancy to seek necessary treatment and the physician's reluctance to refer and thereby restrict potential service delivery.

HMOs/PPOs and Restrictive Access

Armenti (1991) asserted that HMO arrangements for mental health services are the most complex and restrictive in limiting the number of sessions, authorizing visits in smaller "doses" (or with delays and reluctance), requiring more paper-work, having more withholding, and offering lower reimbursement fees. He suggests that PPOs are not as restrictive in this regard. However, many PPO policies restrict access to mental health care by setting benefit maximums so low that the patient is essentially forced to pay the entire cost either through higher percentage copayments or full payment after a small number of treatment sessions has been reached and when therapeutic work remains to be done.

HMOs and other managed care plans effectively restrict services by imposing waiting periods on patients before appointments, requiring completion of an extensive questionnaire, not returning phone calls, and otherwise making use of psychological services difficult or inconvenient (Shulman, 1988). Public complaints about these practices and advocacy by employee groups to employers have started to improve the situation, but there are still far too many instances of this form of service restriction. Just as public concerns over the rising cost of health care brought about the revolution in financing, so too will public concerns about the quality, problems, and effectiveness of this "revolution" produce further changes that benefit patients (Sleek, 1996b). Correspondingly, in our view, this next step will improve the standing of the clinical providers. If the clinician keeps to the "high road" of legitimately advocating on behalf of patients, then regulators and the judiciary will likely resolve conflicts in favor of those patients (which will be concomitantly favorable to clinicians).

Conclusions on Services Restriction

In contrast to our perceptions of a conflict of interest leading to restriction of services, the industry's position is "managed care *when conducted properly* does not restrict care, it eliminates *unnecessary* care and approves payment for clinically necessary care" (Armenti, 1991, p. 125, emphasis added). Perhaps the problems experienced by many patients and clinicians reflect the reality that many managed care entities are *not* conducted properly.

UNDERTREATMENT

Another key element of managed health care is the practice of controlling costs by limiting treatment. Indeed, many managed care companies give financial incentives to their gatekeepers and providers for holding down costs by limiting care. For example, providers in a capitated plan may get bonuses or a share of any profit when annual expenses are less than the amount of money received to administer the benefits. Another method is to "hold back" or "withhold" a part of a payment due a clinician until the end of the year. In this case, the money is given to the clinician only if the plan's budget balances or shows a profit. If the plan runs a deficit, the clinician never receives the money. In both of these situations, the clinician has a direct financial incentive to undertreat, that is, not to provide a needed service in order to keep costs to the plan to a minimum in order to receive more money. Preauthorization by gatekeepers also controls access and use. Armenti (1991) calls these arrangements a "very compelling and seductive economic incentive" (p. 125).

When the gatekeepers for mental health services are the primary care providers, this arrangement can also become a conflict of interest. For instance, when the gatekeeper's share of the company's profit is decreased if expensive services are accessed or when referral is made outside the network, there is a strong financial incentive to limit access or to provide some forms of services that are cheaper (and possibly less effective). Where once a clinician might have advocated for one form of treatment, it may become in his or her financial interest to decide in favor of another treatment modality or approach. While we might hope that practices are dictated by professional standards, placing the gatekeeper in this situation pits the interests of the pocketbook against the interests of the patient. The results of these incentives and restrictions are, as Karen Shore (1996) asserted: "Patients in managed care systems can no longer trust their clinicians' motives, so they must make significant life and death decisions without professional input and support" (p. 324). For example, some pediatric physicians have decided to evaluate and treat childhood disorders themselves, such as ADHD, rather than refer to a psychologist for appropriate evaluation and treatment recommendations. Another incentive to undertreat, however indirectly, is the ever-present threat that the clinician would be terminated from a managed care network if the clinician advocates too often for more sessions and services for patients or regularly exceeds some company limit on number of sessions. The clinician may be labeled "managed care incompatible" and removed from the panel, or may simply no longer receive any referrals from that plan. (This threat is also discussed in the section on "no cause" provisions of managed care contracts.) Certainly the threat to remove the means of earning an income is an incentive to undertreat.

It is the psychologist's ethical obligation to clarify any conflicts of employment or affiliation for the patient's information so that the psychologist can adhere to the APA Ethical Principle 8.03. This obligation includes identifying incentives to undertreat or restrict services.

INFORMATION DISCLOSURE

A number of situations arise in clinical practice within managed care environments in which information is limited or misleading. For example, patients may not be aware of managed care limitations on services covered. Nonetheless, psychologists are bound to practice according to the APA ethical standards. The APA policy statement on managed care articulates, "[P]roviders and patients should be informed of the limitations and restrictions to types and access of psychological services prior to subscribing to a plan (i.e., truth in advertising or explicit statements regarding any financial disincentives to treat and refer patients in need of psychological services)" (Fox, 1989, p. 1024). Thus, provision of information to patients is a professional and ethical duty, whether it is to identify financial disincentives for treatment, to present information about efficacy of treatment and the need for psychotherapy when indicated, to convey facts about insurance or HMO plan coverage for reimbursement of various treatments, or to faithfully portray what a clinician is capable of providing, either by competence or within the limitations of a managed care plan.

Truth in Advertising for the Clinician

The axiom to tell the truth in advertising one's competence or ability to provide services has become more troublesome under the constraints of managed care. Some plans remain in an earlier stance of preferring clinical generalists who can provide a very broad range of services within the managed care framework. Commentators have suggested that managed care seems to prefer those clinicians who charge the least and have less training and lower competence (not those with skill, training, or effectiveness), therefore ensuring that the clinical providers become dependent on the plans (Seligman, 1996; Shore, 1996). Newer behavioral health plans, on the other hand, increasingly attempt to determine what constitutes expertise in certain areas, such as child and adolescent problems or drug and alcohol abuse, and then identify specialists who can provide these services. A recent drive to find specialists in child and family psychology in some areas of the country, for example, developed out of consumer demand for quality services. These developments should help highly qualified clinicians to distinguish themselves from less well-trained or differently qualified providers. We encourage specialty clinicians to educate network managers about what constitutes competence. Such competence may include predoctoral, internship, and postdoctoral experiences related directly to particular problems, treatment techniques, or settings. In the service field for children, adolescents, and families, there are models of training for the clinician to cite in order to establish unique training and skills (e.g., Roberts, Erickson, & Tuma, 1985; Roberts et al., submitted for publication). Additionally, increased efforts to educate clients and the public about the benefits of psychological services from doctoral level clinicians will help in moving employers and managed care corporations to include specialists on their plans and provider networks. Such demonstrations of corporate "caring" and favorable public relations, of course, must be fulfilled in practice, not serve as empty promises.

Clearly, psychiatrists have some advantages by claiming special expertise and abilities in order to receive higher fees. For example, in many, if not most, managed behavioral health care plans, the application sets out a differential fee schedule for psychiatrists, psychologists (e.g., around 82% of psychiatrist's fee), and social workers (e.g., around 63% of psychiatrist's fee). So, too, can the clinician with expertise in child or adolescent psychology describe the advantages to the plan of specialty services (we offer some basic information for the clinician about these in Chapter 7). The clinician should be careful not to overreach in claiming expertise either to a patient or to the plan managers. Although this statement should stand without elaboration, we know of some practitioners who are attempting to capture more clients either as self-payers or through managed care reimbursement by claiming specialty expertise status for a laundry list of problems, situations, and techniques. Should the clinician have special expertise in the child and family area, this should be documented in the application to the panel and in brochures distributed to potential referral sources and clientele.

Clinicians are well advised to identify for *themselves* any financial incentives or disincentives to treat patients' problems in particular ways (Appelbaum, 1993; Newman & Bricklin, 1991). (Incentives to undertreat were discussed in an earlier section.) Obviously, accurate information and communication with the patient is necessary for ethical practice. Participation in a capitated mental health plan particularly opens conflicts of interest for the clinician, and it behooves the clinician to clarify these roles with the patient. We believe that fully informed patients usually select their best options. Ill-informed patients are too often vulnerable to injury in some form; this also opens the clinician to liability suits.

The clinician needs to provide, to the best of his or her ability, accurate information on what services are likely to be covered by a patient's policy or plan. (While we acknowledge that clinicians cannot be responsible for knowing all the nuances of all the plans in one's community, we do urge the responsible clinician to have many of the answers—without the clinician, the patient is likely left without an advocate or source of legitimate information.) In Box 3.1, we give an example of a patient brochure that states that the patient needs to become familiar with his or her particular plan's benefits. However, translation of those policies into real-life practices or providing the questions for the patients to ask of their benefits manager can enhance their ability to understand, request, and get what they need. Before embarking on this, however, the clinician should be familiar with his or her own contract to see if the informational "gag rule" is present (and if so, to determine whether his or her ethical standards and state laws permit the clinician to abide by it).

The clinician needs to clearly indicate to patients which services are not likely to be covered by their plans. Indeed, clinicians can and should still delineate for patients those treatments that are psychologically indicated but for which managed care reimbursement may not be available. Reimbursement

BOX 3.1 SAMPLE STATEMENT ON MEDICAL INSURANCE COVERAGE FOR CLINICIAN'S PRACTICE BROCHURE

Many health insurance policies reimburse the client for the types of psychological services provided by A-1 Clinical Practice. However, the policies may be different in a variety of ways: Some members of the family may be covered and not others; some problems or conditions may be covered and not others; some types of services are covered, and some others are not; some policies set a limit on the number of contacts or sessions for which the patient can be reimbursed; some require that the patient pay a portion or all of the costs and then reimburse the patient for some part of those costs. Although the clinicians in A-1 Clinical Practice are knowledgeable about many of the plans, we advise patients to become familiar with the provisions of their policies.

We have found that the typical insurance plan in this locale will reimburse the patient for (a) individual psychotherapy, (b) group psychotherapy, and less for (c) psychological assessment and test interpretation. Some policies have excluded coverage for (a) marital and family therapy, (b) parent counseling, (c) child counseling, (d) vocational counseling, (e) school-related problems, and (f) court-ordered forensic evaluations. Other policies will reimburse you for expenses for some of these activities only if your primary physician makes a direct request to the managed care plan.

Please note that payment in full is due at the time when services are rendered. Except where required by the managed care plan, A-1 Clinical Practice will not file for reimbursement, although we are happy to provide the documentation necessary for you to file a claim. Health insurance companies should attempt to respond to your needs as a subscriber. However, should you and your insurance carrier have a dispute over a claim, we can only provide information and documentation; negotiating settlement is between you and your company.

A-1 Clinical Practice participates in several managed care plans and health maintenance organizations in this area (e.g., Epitome Health; Apex Behavioral Health Program; ApogeeCare). These plans may require that both we and the patient follow specific procedures. Typically the patient must obtain authorization from the managed care plan to seek services at A-1 Clinical Practice. You will need to consult with your physician or HMO to receive this authorization, which may include a statement authorizing a type of service, any limits on sessions, and possibility of extension. If prior authorization is required and you do not obtain that authorization, the charge for services will be your responsibility.

> All charges incurred are ultimately your responsibility. These include any copayments required by your insurance company or managed care plan, payments for services not covered under the plan, lengthy telephone consultations, or missed sessions. Should you have any questions about your treatment, the charges, or the insurance/HMO coverage, the clinicians and staff of A-1 Clinical Practice will be happy to discuss them with you.
>
> In order for us to provide the information necessary for the insurance companies or managed care plans, you will need to sign a form authorizing A-1 Clinical Practice to send the requested information and answer inquiries (both telephoned and written) about these diagnostic and therapeutic activities. Most insurance companies and managed care firms attempt to respect privacy and maintain confidentiality of records of its enrollees. However, in providing information necessary for clients to be reimbursed, A-1 Clinical Practice cannot make any assurances about how that information will be used or who will have access to it.

policies notwithstanding, the clinician is professionally obligated to outline what services are needed. Additionally, information for special appeal or advocacy may be needed by the patient (such as in a case where referral outside the network may be necessary).

Truth in Advertising for Managed Care

Several commentators have noted that managed care thrives on patient ignorance or disempowerment (Shore, 1996). It is in both the clinician's and the patient's best interest to have adequate information available for decision-making. However, just as we think the professionals who provide services should practice "truth in advertising," so, too, do we think that the managed care companies should be held to the same standard. Fully informed consumers can make the best decisions. There are too few regulations in many states governing the practices of managed care entities. This situation seems to be changing; state and federal laws, insurance regulations, and court decrees are adding more requirements of full and complete provision of information about coverage, exclusions, limitations, rights, and appeal processes. These changes seem inevitably to benefit those enrolled in the plans and, consequently, those who provide the services within the plans. For example, Massachusetts state law now bars managed care companies from limiting clinicians from providing full information to a patient (including discussion about treatment not covered under a patient's plan).

"Gag Rules"

Although many managed care companies deny their existence, contracts between managed care companies and providers often have clauses that limit what a clinician can tell the patient (or may be interpreted as such). Typically, limitations are placed on telling patients about alternative treatments, the need for additional treatment, or the limits placed on the provider for certain treatments for the patient. These "gag rules" imposed by managed care companies have been challenged in the lay press, in the U.S. Congress and state legislatures, and in the courts. A managed care contract might have a clause or wording such as, "The clinician agrees not to disparage the health care plan or its procedures, policies, or personnel to any person, including enrollees in the plan or other providers. Disparagement of the plan will be considered administrative noncompliance and the clinician may be subject to dismissal." Another gag clause might read: "Clinicians shall make no statements or communications that might be construed to undermine the confidence of the plan's enrollees, the employers, or the public in the health care corporation or in the quality of care that enrollees might receive."

Gag rules have a chilling effect on the clinician who is attempting to practice in a professional manner when providing adequate information and services to the patient. Such gag rules have been forced on psychologists and other mental health providers in managed care plans. Some limits on communication about treatment have been modified (after public pressure) in some parts of the country (Sleek, 1995, 1996b), yet the implication is always present that a clinician may be dropped from a panel without cause or due process should he or she advocate for a patient too strongly or provide too much information such that the patient demands and receives expensive services within or outside the network (Shore, 1996; Wooley, 1993). In several states, laws prohibit "gag" provisions in provider contracts over communicating certain information (Sleek, 1996c).

LIABILITY AND "HOLD HARMLESS" CLAUSES

The changes in practice arrangements resulting from managed care agreements have further complicated the liability situation. Depending on the contract clause, the clinician is usually responsible for acquiring and maintaining adequate malpractice or liability insurance (usually a stated minimum such as $1 million) when offering services through a network or panel. The contract forms typically ask for evidence of such liability insurance.

Another contract clause that creates difficulties for the clinician's liability has been the "hold harmless" provision. These provisions usually distance the clinician from the managed care corporation in cases where negligence is claimed against the clinician as a provider of services. These clauses protect the managed care entity and place the clinician in potential jeopardy. That is, the "hold harmless" provision may state that the provider will hold the managed care corporation harmless in any malpractice or liability litigation (or otherwise "indemnify" the organization). How this can be interpreted adversely to the clinician is that the service provider is responsible for the services, even when instructed or restricted by the managed care company personnel or policies that such services will not be reimbursed. Thus, the clinician could be responsible and liable for actions taken by the managed care organization without decision-making input into what those actions might be and potentially without even being allowed to discuss it fully with the patient (e.g., to restrict the number of sessions or to disallow certain services from coverage). The clinician clearly should be agreeable to liability for his or her own actions in providing the service, but the "hold harmless" clause seemingly makes him or her responsible for the managed care entity's decisions as well. Accountability seems proper when clinicians are responsible for their own clinical decision-making and treatment actions, not when the decisions are taken out of their hands by a managed care gatekeeper or review authority.

A California court decision (*Wickline v. State of California*) established a legal precedent that insurers, HMOs, and other managed care entities can be held liable for harm when their cost-containment procedures lead to patient injury. Prior to this case, the "hold harmless" clauses and prevailing notions held that only the providers of services themselves were responsible. The *Wickline* case established that the third-party payer (viz, insurer or managed care company) is responsible for its negligence in policies and actions (e.g., premature termination of treatment, negligent gatekeeping decisions, poor credentialing; see Newman, 1995). *Wickline* also established the standards by extension from medical to psychological services that the clinician is responsible for protesting the payer's denial of treatment or recommendation for length of treatment. If the clinician does not protest, preferably in writing, he or she may be held liable for the treatment termination decision. When the clinician formally protests, he or she still does not avoid total responsibility for treatment of the patient, but presumably shares in the responsibility for premature termination of treatment with the managed care entity (Newman & Bricklin, 1991), and a better case may be made for the managed care company assuming the majority of the liability. A later court case, *Wilson v. Blue Cross of Southern California*, established that the provider does not have to protest a managed care decision in order to get the entity's liability involved. However, the clinician still bears some responsibility for treatment actions (e.g., premature termination).

The clinician is advised to examine carefully the wording of any "hold harmless" or indemnification provisions in managed care contracts. Poor or ambiguous wording could leave one open to liability even when the HMO or PPO policies might be faulty (Higuchi, 1994). Consultation with an attorney or with the clinician's state professional association can help clarify these clauses.

There are other cases currently in the courts that may ultimately find that practices accepted by managed care companies today are negligent and that providers are therefore subject to legal and financial liability. Thus, it is mandatory that providers working in a managed care environment strive to balance quality with cost containment, abide by professional standards and ethical guidelines, and maintain the quality of their care above all. Although sometimes difficult, it is not impossible in most cases to provide quality care that is also cost-effective.

The clinician's liability is always related to conformity to a recognized standard of care. A commentator on legal and ethical issues in managed care practice has warned that, as the changes in mental health practice fostered by managed care reimbursement policies become widely accepted, these changed practices will become the "legitimate standards of care" (Appelbaum, 1993). This will pose further dilemmas and challenges for those who wish to practice differently, yet competently, but are apparently forced to accept the managed care philosophy in order to provide services to those in need.

APPEALING ADVERSE COVERAGE DECISIONS

Surveys of private practitioners reveal many reported problems of getting extensions to a set number of sessions or coverage of a disallowed presenting problem or treatment procedure (APA Practice Directorate, 1996; Bowers & Knapp, 1993; Sinnett & Holen, 1993). If, as suggested in the preceding section, the clinician is at least partially responsible not only for his or her own treatment decisions but also for those made by the managed care entity (under the *Wickline* ruling), then it is clear that clinicians *must* appeal adverse decisions made by the corporate staff or protocol. This obligation to appeal derives from two important rationales:

- Clinicians must advocate for what is best for their patients, despite disincentives or obstacles for such advocacy. This is an ethical and moral obligation of professionalism.
- Clinicians must establish a record of having appealed adverse treatment decisions to protect themselves in cases of potential liability. This is a necessary self-protection strategy.

Some provider contracts require the clinician to renounce the right of appeal of claims for benefits or coverage on behalf of a patient (Wright, 1992).

Such clauses place clinicians in jeopardy and should be challenged. The clinician who advocates for patients vis à vis managed care faces the potential of being dropped from a panel for being "incompatible with managed care" (Fox, 1995; Shore, 1996; Wooley, 1993). Many provider contracts contain clauses allowing termination of the provider from the panel/network without cause, thus denying any appeals or due process procedures. Through these "no-cause" provisions, the corporation can terminate the contract without having to justify its actions, which can be used to punish "troublemaking" clinicians. In 1996, the New Jersey Psychological Association filed a complaint against a large behavioral health care corporation, stating that the "no-cause" termination clause and actions are harmful. The complaint alleges that psychologists were dropped from the corporation's network by designating them "not managed care compatible" ("New Jersey Psychologists," 1996, p. 11). The corporation took this termination action presumably because the psychologists sought to use more sessions than authorized (even though the number of sessions did not exceed the patients' benefits packages). These "no-cause" terminations are a very real threat to the clinician who advocates for his or her patients, but they do not obviate professional and ethical responsibility to act in the patient's best interests. These issues have not been fully litigated. The New Jersey action may be a critical case for determining the clinician's ethical/legal duties. Higuchi (1994) outlined several steps for the clinician to take when terminated without cause. These include:

- Become knowledgeable about contract provisions regarding termination.
- Ascertain if the company followed its own procedures.
- In a cordial discussion with staff of the organization (provider relations officer), ask about procedures for getting reinstated and what will happen with the care of the clinician's patients currently being served.
- If not reinstated on appeal, the clinician might consider lodging a written complaint with details on actions, practices, and competence. The clinician should keep notes (dates, names, and content of conversations) and documentation in case of later litigation. The clinician will have a better case if he or she were "punished" by termination because the clinician's actions were on behalf of a patient in need (e.g., appealing an adverse treatment decision as called for in competent practice, legal case law, and the profession's ethical standards).

TREATMENT BEYOND REIMBURSEMENT

Upon failing to gain approval for extension of coverage for further treatment sessions, the clinician and patient are faced with the dilemma of terminating therapy at that point, referring to another clinician or service, or continuing treatment under an arrangement of fully self-paying, pro bono (donated) services or reduced fee-for-service. While the clinician clearly has an obligation to the patient under his or her care, serving too many patients essentially for free would eventually bankrupt the ethical clinician (and patients would not be well-served in this situation).

Some clinicians have resolved this dilemma by putting treatments "on hold" once the annual limits on number of sessions are reached. For example, one appalled commentator quoted another clinician's joke that she had entered the season of clinicians and patients saying, "Well so long—see you next year" (Wooley, 1993, p. 393). Yet for many, this may be an unfortunate reality. Wooley also cited another treatment center practice of sending telegrams to managed care corporations when requests are denied for extension of benefits. These telegrams notify the corporation that at specified time and date, the client will become the corporation's "legal and medical responsibility" (p. 393). This action usually prompts the corporation to extend benefits out of fear of liability.

Clinicians are under ethical and professional practice obligations to avoid abandoning patients. Failure to provide services to the level of the recognized standard of care is unethical and opens the clinician to liability. When managed care seeks its cost savings by premature termination or limitation on sessions, then this issue becomes most salient. This is a dilemma because managed care attempts to shift the legal responsibility to the clinician to provide the necessary care, even if not reimbursed, and the clinician must not abandon patients in need. As noted earlier, the clinician needs to establish a record of having appealed the decision, but he or she also must avoid the perception of having dropped a patient because coverage is limited (Resnick, Bottinelli, Puder-York, Harris, & O'Keefe, 1994). Consequently, the clinician needs to provide for an adequately planned termination. A written plan, provided to the patient, will benefit both the patient and the clinician. Furthermore, the clinician is well advised to provide from the outset full information about the limitations of coverage, the possible disruption of the therapeutic relationship, and the eventual termination process. Clearly the situation and status of a patient will affect whether the clinician continues treatment beyond the approved or reimbursed number of sessions. A clinician who is treating an adolescent boy who is suicidal or a girl who is anorexic and acutely harmful to herself will recognize the obligation to continue treatment until remedies can be found. Nonemergency situations usually are less amenable to appeal for continued coverage from the managed care entity so the clinician may indeed be obligated to provide the necessary care, or an appropriate referral. Appelbaum (1993) suggested:

> As has always been the case when insurance benefits expired and patients could not or would not assume responsibility for the costs

of care, clinicians' obligations are limited to referral (if free or low-cost care is available) or appropriate termination. Depending on the length of time that therapy has gone on, termination may require from one to several sessions to wrap up and consolidate the gains of treatment.... No more can be reasonably required, although it is noteworthy that this is another issue that the courts have yet to address. (p. 254)

CONFIDENTIALITY

A major concern of health care providers (and their patients) is the transfer of information about the patient's condition and treatment to third parties. Although confidentiality of psychologist–patient communications is respected in most state laws, there have been an increased number of exceptions to this patient privilege (such as in the case of suspected child/elder abuse and vocalized specific threats to self or others). One more exception, but one that the patient explicitly must authorize, is documentation of problems, diagnosis, and treatment when third parties are asked to pay for services. Thus, in order for the clinician to provide the necessary information to insurance companies or managed care plans, the patient (parent/guardian/enrollee/subscriber) needs to sign a consent statement or special form authorizing the release of information to the managed care company. This consent to release information should also cover answers to inquiries (both telephoned and written) about diagnostic and therapeutic activities. The information eventually requested by the managed care company may vary from minimal to comprehensive. The requests may be simply for documentation (with diagnosis and treatment plan) or a review process after the fact or sometimes in an appeal for extended coverage of sessions. The legality of these consents to release all information requested by a insurer, even when fully informed, have not been established. Furthermore, the APA Ethical Principles state that psychologists should not release information to unqualified persons.

Although most insurance companies and managed care firms attempt to respect privacy and maintain confidentiality of records of their enrollees, there are few effective controls. Some state laws and insurance regulations outline what can be requested and provided, yet too many instances are known of violations of confidential records to claim otherwise (e.g., see Higuchi, 1994). Relevant to this point, one of us (MCR) once had a patient's father, whose job was overseeing the health benefits for a major company, pay cash out of his pocket rather than have his family's information bandied about the system. He said he knew how lax the procedures were in his office. Concerns for confidentiality and loss of privacy in the managed care environment have always ranked high among surveys of psychologists (Bowers & Knapp, 1993; Sinnett & Holen, 1993). Some clinicians refuse to sign managed care contracts because of concerns over the lack of confidentiality and what problems that lack causes in the therapeutic relationship. Some managed care companies routinely review a random sample of charts for procedural documentation, and providers can be terminated if they do not allow a representative of the managed care firm to read and/or copy those charts. Patients rarely know this may happen when they access their mental health benefits.

As with most aspects of managed care, the clinician serves the patient best by providing information about the limits of confidentiality, especially when the patient is seeking reimbursement for payments. We recommend something like the statements made in Box 3.1 and Box 3.2. Additionally, the clinician should discuss the information transfer with the patient from the outset. Informed consent is the rule; the clinician must respect the patient's decision to release the information in order to receive reimbursement.

MANAGED CARE CONTRACTS

All of the potential ethical and legal issues discussed thus far come to the forefront when the clinician considers signing a contract with a managed care company. The clinician should remember that contracts are legally binding documentation of a business relationship. As in all business contracts, the clinician is well advised to consult an attorney with expertise in health care contracts. The clinician may seek other sources for reviewing contracts (e.g., Giles, 1993; Higuchi, 1994; Richardson & Austad, 1991).

It is critically important for the clinician to read each managed care contract carefully before signing. There are substantial differences between managed care contracts, including differences in fees, terms, financial arrangements, and provider liability. Capitated contracts can be even trickier, as the clinician or group must determine (or estimate) in advance the volume of patients that might access services and the likelihood of those patients using a particular service (number and frequency of visits). If the clinician is a specialist (such as a child clinical psychologist), the regular formula the company uses to determine the rate of visits may not apply. In the following sections we highlight a number of issues the clinician should consider when reviewing a managed care contract.

Information about the Company

The clinician is advised to request information about the managed care organization, such as the number of covered lives, how many children are members,

---

**BOX 3.2. SAMPLE STATEMENT OF
CONFIDENTIALITY FOR THE
CLINICIAN'S PRACTICE BROCHURE**

A-1 Clinical Practice respects the privacy and confidentiality of information provided by the children and families served to the extent possible under law. One specific situation in which this commitment to confidentiality may be broken is when you request reimbursement from your insurance company, HMO, or other managed care policy for payments to A-1 Clinical Practice. That is, when you ask your health care policy to pay for the services, you are giving permission for us to provide information requested by the insurance company or review panel. This information may include diagnostic or treatment information. A-1 Clinical Practice cannot determine how that information is used or who reviews that information once it leaves our office. Sometimes the full clinical record will be requested. Some of the information may be computerized and placed in a databank accessible to many others. We cannot assume any responsibility for the information once it leaves our office. Basic information is required on the claim form you will sign. If additional information beyond what the clinician feels is reasonable is requested, we will inform you of what is needed and review with you what will be provided. Remember, it is your decision to file for payment of these services; we will honor that decision, but will have to comply with the regulations to the best of our legal and ethical responsibilities.

Footnote: The clinician's brochure for new patients should also contain information on other limiting aspects of therapeutic confidentiality, such as "clear and present danger" to self or others, child abuse or elder abuse, attorney/collection agency arrangements, or court subpoena.

---

and which local employers/companies offer this managed care plan exclusively, and which offer it as an option. A copy of the plan's benefit package would be useful for understanding how it informs its enrollees. Consulting with other colleagues, the clinician can determine the general reputation of the organization in terms of its ethics, payment history, quality programming, number of panelists, and annual turnover rate of staff and providers. (Turnover in staff that exceeds 15–20% may signal a need for caution.) Financial stability is critically important as managed care companies emerge and flounder or are merged with and absorbed by other companies. Financial reports are available, and it is essential that the clinician keep up to date on the financial status of all contracted companies even after signing. As previously stated, states do not provide a safety net for HMOs, so companies can and do go bankrupt, resulting in providers not being paid and patients not being served. With current information on the financial status of the organization, the clinician will be in a better position to get out of a situation that looks like potential financial failure, or at least to limit losses. Information on a managed care firm's financial resources is available through the state's insurance commission or by reading A. M. Best Company's books (which review insurance companies) periodically. The clinician should also determine if there is any litigation involving the company as well. If the organization is a new one, there may be little track record, but the clinician can learn about the company's stated philosophies through its literature and something about what it will be like through the reputations of the new leadership and staff. The more the clinician knows about a company, the better informed will be the decision about signing with it.

If the clinician wants to negotiate changes in a contract, this may be a possibility. If the clinician is a specialist the company needs, or if he or she has a particularly good reputation or is in great demand in the community, he or she may have more success in negotiating changes in standard contracts. However, the managed care company may deny any and all requested changes to the contract. At that point, the clinician must decide whether the contract can be accepted as it is, what the risks are, and what other options may be present.

The clinician needs to remember that contracts he or she signs are legal documents that obligate the provider to specific duties. The clinician, considering an invitation to join a managed care provider panel, must be certain that he or she has a full understanding of the contract and all of its provisions before signing. It is advisable to seek the consultation of an attorney in any uncertain situations. In order to decrease attorney fees, some local psychological associations or practice groups maintain a relationship with an attorney, usually one familiar with both mental health and managed care, to review all contracts for the group. Since it is likely that many providers will be reviewing the same contracts, this can reduce the cost for everyone and provide the strength in numbers often needed to negotiate changes in contracts with managed care companies.

Covered Services

The clinician needs to review what services are covered and what are excluded by the plan. For example, educational testing, including testing and treatment of attention deficits, may be specifically excluded. If the clinician's specialty is ADHD, this may not be the right plan for contracting. The clinician should also determine what copayments and deductibles patients will have to pay. In many cases, this will be an overwhelming task, such as when a large managed care company negotiates individualized contracts with many employers in a locale. However, at a minimum, the clinician should request the basic or standard deductible and copayment schedules. If the company later offers modified plans to other employers, the clinician should ensure that the contract does not obligate him or her to accept later revisions and should receive updates in advance when contracts with employers change or are added.

Payments to Providers

Payment to the clinician may be at a discounted rate (from his or her usual charges), a standard fee established by the managed care organization, or a decreasing fee when the number of sessions rises. The clinician needs to determine how the fee rates are set and what influences them. The clinician should also check to see that the contract requires the plan to make payment within a specific number of days (usually 30–45) and that there are provisions for penalties and interest on late payments from the plan. (Deferred/late payments often seemed to be the norm for some managed care plans; this may be another action to slow down cash flow or "punish" the troublemaking clinicians who advocate for their patients or a sign of the plan's financial instability.) One of us (LKH) has had several bad experiences with this issue. First, one managed care organization has taken an excessive amount of time to pay several claims. Even when reminded of their contractual obligation to pay the full fee (due to delayed payment), it was difficult and sometimes impossible to collect. In a second case, a managed care organization routinely paid only a small portion of the amount due, but claimed that the 30-day provision did not apply if *any* payment, even if incorrect, had been made within the 30-day limit. In this case, it was not possible to collect the balance. However, the provider had the option of resigning from the plan.

Withholds

Many plans withhold a certain percent of a clinician's discounted payment against future services, referrals, and hospitalizations. (These are often the "holdbacks" used by a capitated plan in case of budget overruns.) Details on the formula for the withholds and how the funds are managed and released can be obtained from the plan manager. Some clinicians may be grouped for comparison with others who are similar or dissimilar, or the withhold rate could be based on each clinical provider's individual performance. Any withhold amounts should be described on the Explanation of Benefits (EOB) the clinician will receive along with the payment. Documentation could help in the recovery of any withholds due at the end of the period.

Liability Insurance Requirements

The contract may set a minimum amount of liability insurance the clinician is required to carry. If it is more than the current coverage, the clinician needs to determine whether the referrals from the plan are worth the increased premium, especially given the discounted fees.

Preauthorization and UR

The clinician will need to find out what type of authorization is needed to begin treatment with a patient, how often reauthorization is required, and what the procedure is for reviews of utilization. Contract phrases to look for are "prior authorization," "concurrent review," and "retrospective reviews." The clinician can ask for a list of those who serve on the review panel in order to determine their qualifications. The written rules for reviews should be available to all providers. The clinician will want to know what procedures are used to ensure confidentiality during the review periods and what information gets computerized (in order to be knowledgeable for the patient who will inquire). The clinician should determine what the appeal process is and who (qualifications) handles appeals. A noteworthy element might be whether the clinician can request a "like provider" as the appeal gatekeeper (e.g., a licensed child psychologist). Alternatively, the company may reserve the right to designate the appeal agent for all appeals (e.g., the company "house psychiatrist"). Some of these elements may be mandated by state laws. "Quality assurance" clauses should be clarified through questions such as: How are these reviews or surveys conducted? Who is responsible for gathering patient satisfaction and outcome data? How is this information used?

Referrals

The clinician needs to be informed about provisions for making referrals. The clinician should inquire about whether the patient needs to be referred back to the primary care provider for subsequent mental health referrals, whether the clinician can refer the patient directly to other providers, and whether the clinician can refer the patient out of the plan's network. (Some plans require the provider to assume financial responsibility for any referrals outside the network. If so, this needs to be known well in advance.)

"No Disparagement" Clause

These "gag" provisions are generally unacceptable because they prevent the clinician from abiding by the Ethical Principles. These clauses are becoming less prevalent, but may appear in various forms.

"Hold Harmless" Clause

As noted earlier, some plans require that the clinician accept all malpractice risks and hold the company completely harmless. This clause could make the clinician liable for treatment and referral decisions made by the managed care company. If the company will not remove the clause, then the *Wickline* case makes it important for the clinician to appeal adverse treatment decisions and document them. The clinician may have limited protection if he or she is in a group that spreads the risk by having a committee decide on referrals and hospitalizations. However, he or she may still be held liable for treatment decisions. (Obviously this clause interacts with how appeals can be made and whether the clinician can be threatened with termination from the provider panel for advocating too much for patients). The clinician also needs to determine if his or her insurance carrier will cover the practice if the "hold harmless" clause remains in the contract. An agreeable contract might be for both the managed care organization and the clinical provider to indemnify each other such that the organization is responsible for its own negligence, but not the clinician's, and the clinician is responsible for his or her own negligence, but not that of the organization. It is recommended that clinicians seek legal advice when such issues arise.

Hospitalization

If a patient needs to be hospitalized and the clinician does not have privileges at the plan's contracted hospitals, what arrangements can be made for the patient? Will the clinician need to turn over care to another provider? Can the patient be admitted to one of the hospitals at which the clinician does have privileges? Or, can the clinician be granted temporary privileges at one of the plan hospitals? The plan's back-up coverage provisions for crisis or emergency situations should also be identified.

Confidentiality of Records

To protect confidentiality, the contract should provide for the managed care company's access to the patient's records only with the patient/legal guardian's written permission. In reality, by their nature and procedures, most managed care plans ignore confidentiality. Nonetheless, the clinician can try to negotiate for the best protection possible for the patient. As noted, the clinician needs to determine the qualifications of the person who will be reviewing clinical information. An understanding of the reviewer's ethical commitment to confidentiality can be determined in order to help the clinician explain the process to the patient. The clinician might also ask how they will use the information in making treatment authorization decisions. If the information requested seems excessive at some point, the clinician may need to speak with the person's supervisor to determine whether the detailed information requested is really necessary. If the clinician determines that providing the information will violate his or her ethical and professional obligations to the patient, the clinician may need to discuss with the patient the company's request for information, discuss the likely outcome that the company may not approve services without the information, and jointly agree with the patient on what both will do. The patient must ultimately make the decision on release of records, but we feel this should be a well-informed decision.

Continuity of Care

The clinician will need to know what will happen if the covered person's benefit plan (child patient or parent as plan enrollee) is changed or terminated. The plan should outline any provisions for continuing care. What is the clinician's liability for those patients? Abandonment presents a serious legal and ethical problem. The clinician should be aware that reducing fees to continue treatment of someone whose benefits have expired for the year may also affect the reimbursement level when the benefits are reinstated the following year. Clinicians report both good and bad experiences when employers change managed care organizations during treatment. For example, one company allowed anyone who had started treatment a 6-month period to complete it and paid the clinicians' full fees if they were not contracted providers with the new company. However, another company allowed a maximum of two visits to terminate or transfer care to one of the new plan's providers.

Termination of the Contract

The contract should allow the clinician to terminate the business relationship within a reasonable amount of time if it becomes unsuitable. Although a long-term contract may sound good, the health care market is constantly changing, and the clinician may find that he or she wants to be relieved of any obligations to a certain managed care company before the contract period is up. Failure to reimburse the clinician within a reasonable time after service delivery should be cause for termination of the contract by the provider.

Termination by the Managed Care Company

Contracts should allow the managed care company to terminate a business relationship with a provider—that is only fair. However, this termination should be done only with "cause" and following some explicit "due process" procedure. "No-cause" terminations are unacceptable. Termination "for cause" should require a written explanation from the organization detailing its justification. The contract may contain provisions about continuation or termination in the case of a change in corporate structure (merger or buy-out). The appeals procedures should be clearly stated.

Provider Directory

Sometimes a plan may list all the providers in a directory including name and specialty. As a clinical child/pediatric psychologist, for example, the clinician might be listed in a less crowded category, a distinct advantage in most cases. The clinician might ask to review the listing before it is published.

Additional Documents

If any other documents or forms are mentioned in a contract (peer review procedures, grievance procedures, etc.) the clinician should insist on receiving a copy of each additional document prior to signing the contract.

Other Questionable Provisions

Some additional contract clauses should be questioned by the clinician if present:

- "Exclusivity": The clinician may sign away the ability to contract with any other organizations. This is inadvisable because clinicians need flexibility and should not be forced to rely on referrals from only one company.
- "No competition": The clinician may agree that he or she will not compete with the organization in providing services for a number of years after termination in the same area as the organization. The clinician must consider such provisions and their potential impact carefully.

Exclusion from PPO Panels

Because courts generally consider PPOs to be procompetitive by nature, it is difficult to challenge a decision of a PPO to refuse an application from a prospective provider. Therefore, "restraint of trade" claims against PPOs are usually unsuccessful. However, Higuchi (1994) proposes six steps psychologists should take if their applications to PPO panels are denied:

1 | Get the specific reasons for the refusal in writing. This can help with devising a new strategy for reapplying.

2 | Determine whether the PPO is rejecting all psychologists' applications or whether they have met their quota for psychologists. If all psychologist applications are being rejected, the prospective applicant should check their state's PPO law to determine whether it contains a "willing provider" provision (many states do). This concept basically means that all providers with the necessary credentials must be added to the provider panel if they request it. If there is a willing provider law, it will probably protect psychologists as a class of health care provider, even though it may not guarantee that any individual will be accepted.

3 | If state law does not require that the PPO allow psychologists to serve on panels, the decision is usually left to the managed care organization. In that case, the psychologist should try to maintain a good relationship with the PPO while negotiating a satisfactory resolution. This will benefit all parties, including the patient; a hostile relationship will benefit no one.

4 | Determine whether the state PPO law has a requirement that the PPO cover services by a nonpreferred provider if an enrollee seeks their services. If the law requires that such services be covered, even though it may also allow for higher copayments or deductibles, the psychologist will have a good case for getting services covered if the PPO is not in compliance with state law.

5 | Determine whether the psychologist's services are subject to ERISA provisions since ERISA plans are generally exempt from state laws.

6 | If the psychologist believes that a specific PPO discriminates against psychologists as a class, Higuchi (1994) encourages clinicians to contact the APA's Legal and Regulatory Affairs Division, Office of Managed Care, for assistance.

With any of these issues, the clinician can generally contact either their state psychological association or the APA for information and guidance.

CONCLUDING REMARKS

There are controls in place in most managed care programs that help to minimize some of the more negative features of managed care. Managed care companies are attempting to gather more objective data on providers, and credentialing tends to be an ongoing rather than a one-time process. However, large mental health managed care entities tend to look at their largest providers (those with the most patients) for comparison, so specialty providers are less likely to be included. Data on child mental health usage is also less likely to be available. Quality assurance and utilization review, provider credentialing, medical records reviews, customer satisfaction ratings, and customer grievance procedures can help ensure that quality is maintained, when the information is used appropriately. Within psychology, professional standards, ethical principles, and the risk of malpractice suits may also prevent those provider behaviors that adversely affect quality (Newman & Bricklin, 1991). State laws are constantly changing and generally are requiring managed care companies to be more responsible and to protect patients' rights. In addition, some protections for providers are also being written into law.

We caution that we are not attorneys. What we have recommended here is our perception of best practice. Varying state laws and different managed care practices and contracts make the issues of legality more complex than we can elucidate here. The clinician's state or local psychological association may have an attorney available who is knowledgeable about mental health law and practice within managed care environments. If not, the clinician is advised to consult an attorney over these issues. The Practice Directorate of the APA maintains a Legal and Regulatory Affairs Office (202-336-5886) with an Office of Managed Care for consultation to members on the complexity of relationships between psychological health care providers and managed care entities. The Practice Directorate also provides basic information through its FAXcess service (dial 508-230-2049 from a fax machine and follow instructions on how to access the documents). Document topics include a "checklist of common managed care provider contract provisions," "insuring your office practice," and "what to include in a managed care proposal," among others. Similarly, the clinician can access Practice Directorate information through the APA's home page on the World Wide Web (http://www.apa.org).

Of course, what does not change across the states or managed care organizations is the clinician's allegiance to ethical and competent practice. In order to assist patients maximally and to protect the clinician's practice, we advise the refrain of "document, document, document." The clinician, attempting to practice ethically and competently, needs to recognize that documentation and justification of psychological services are not just onerous and intrusive, but important facts of business life. Psychologists are necessarily held as accountable for their treatments as is everybody else who offers services or products. We hold ourselves to no less than we hold other providers of services.

Adapting to the Managed Care Environment

A psychologist was contacted by the mother of a child to arrange for an evaluation and possible treatment of the child's increasing difficulties with school, peers, and low self-esteem. The mother informed the psychologist that she had spoken with the intake coordinator at her managed care company, who did a 15-minute phone interview. The mother also informed the psychologist that she now had authorization for one additional therapy session. After a session with the child's parents, the psychologist called the HMO to request that additional sessions be authorized. She was told that the intake coordinator had performed the single authorized 90801 intake assessment by phone and that the psychologist would have to bill the session (which was with the parents only) as a 90844 individual therapy visit and *must* provide a diagnosis based on that visit, even though at that point no providers had actually met with the child. The psychologist protested, but was informed that without a diagnosis, the session would not be paid for by the managed care company, and no more sessions would be approved.

Adapting to the managed care environment presents many challenges. Clinicians must be well-informed regarding the contracts they have signed and the procedures they must follow with each company with whom they have contracted and must be knowledgeable regarding outcome measures and how they can be used (and misused). They may face road blocks and obstacles in trying to join managed care panels and in trying to advocate for and with their patients. In this chapter, we will address these issues and provide suggestions for the clinician who wishes to practice within a managed care environment.

ACCESSING PROVIDER PANELS GENERALLY

Many managed care companies initially filled their panels of providers with clinicians who indicated they were able to cover a wide range of patient ages and problems. This early panel loading of generalists allowed companies to publicize their ability to provide diverse services to their enrollees. Furthermore, the companies would, in their view, need fewer clinicians in total because, presumably, all necessary services and competencies were represented by generalist clinicians. Thus, there was a presumption that "one size clinician fits all needs."

Many clinicians with specialty backgrounds in child and family problems redefined themselves as generalists in order to contract with the managed care companies. While feeling the pressure to do this disgruntled many who had sought out and completed specialty training, other clinicians perceived that survival depended on it. The disgruntlement increased on all sides over time: The child specialist clinician often had to take referrals of patients for whom specialty skills were irrelevant, generalist clinicians were receiving child and family referrals for whom their skills were undeveloped or inappropriate, and employers and managed care organizations received complaints about inadequate services.

Although a shift to greater specificity of skills and abilities has emerged to some degree, provider panels remain mostly generalists. At least one well-placed commentator on managed care trends, Nicholas Cummings (1996), has emphasized that specialization is not compatible with a future in managed care. Consequently, the child-oriented clinician may wish to be listed as a generalist in order to maximize patient referrals, if his or her background can support such a claim. (Indeed, many child clinicians were trained in general clinical techniques in adult-oriented programs, with the child specialty work "added on" as extra courses and practicum experiences.)

Armenti (1991) states that certain clinician characteristics are preferred by managed care panels: clinicians with experience in "Mental Health *and* Substance Abuse Training and Experience, Ability to Render Emergency and Crisis Intervention Services, Behaviorally Trained, Uses Community Resources, Member of a Group Practice, and Community Mental Health Center or Agency Background" (p. 123).

As we noted in the chapter on ethical and legal issues (Chapter 3), prior to signing a contract with a managed care company, a clinician will want to know as much about the company as possible: how large their patient base is, which employers offer their plan, financial strength, the experiences of other psychologists working with the company in terms of difficulty getting approval for treatment or assessment or collecting payment, and type and amount of precertification and UR required. All of these issues may impact the clinician's decision regarding joining their panel.

Assuming the clinician decides he or she wants to join their panel, there are different ways to approach the company. If the panel is currently "open" (accepting new applications from all providers), the clinician can call the provider relations department and ask for an application. A cover letter should be included with the application indicating that the clinician is applying to be a provider and clearly stating one's area(s) of expertise, if appropriate. If the clinician wants to be identified as a specialist (e.g., having greater than average specialty skills in clinical child or pediatric psychology), he or she should be certain that the specialty is noted in every blank asking for such information. Specialty skills should be highlighted and repeated often throughout the application.

If the clinician is uncertain whether a provider panel is open (or has been told it is closed), he or she will need to take a more aggressive approach by sending unsolicited information. It is the applicant's job to sell the company on his/her services in the introductory letter and materials. See the sample letter in Box 4.1 for an example of a cover letter requesting an application. This is where the clinician with unique qualifications or specialty skills might have an advantage over the generalist clinician. When panels are closed because of too many providers with the same credentials, then marketing one's special abilities should be carefully approached. For example, if the clinician were fluent in Spanish or American Sign Language and these skills were important for the population served by a managed care organization, an application might be accepted. Similarly, as detailed in the next section, specialty credentials in child, adolescent, family, or pediatric psychology offer an advantage in gaining access to a provider panel.

If encouraged to do so by the provider relations representative, the clinician may want to include data on utilization or customer satisfaction from his or her practice. Means and standard deviations should be provided along with sample data collection forms, if appropriate. Such information demonstrates that the clinician is serious and well-informed about the managed care company's need for such information. If the clinician has not collected practice data of this type, he or she should indicate a willingness to collect these data, perhaps using the managed care company's tools. In addition to customer satisfaction forms, it is helpful to describe the clinician's methods of collecting outcome data with children. Currently, most managed care companies do not have specialized forms or data collection procedures for children, so demonstrating that the clinician can collect quantifiable data from children is likely to be impressive.

It is important for the clinician to follow up with phone calls after sending unsolicited letters or applications. The clinician should ask if the representative has had an opportunity to read the letter and whether he or she has any questions. If so, they should be addressed as succinctly as possible, providing detail only as requested. If the representative seems interested, the clinician should ask what more information would be needed in order to be added to their panel. Even if

BOX 4.1. SAMPLE LETTER TO MANAGED CARE COMPANY REQUESTING AN APPLICATION

February 20, 1997

Mr. James Black
Managed Care Company B
1 Healthcare Drive
Anytown, Anystate

Dear Mr. Black:

As you are aware, Anytown has a population of 300,000 people, and approximately one third of them are children or adolescents. Of these 100,000 or so children and adolescents, it is estimated that up to 20% will have a diagnosable mental disorder. As a clinical child psychologist, I have the training and experience to quickly and efficiently diagnose and treat many of the mental health problems these children present. I noticed from reading your provider list that you do not currently have any child specialists on your psychology panel. Because your company insures employees of the city, the school district, and several other local employers, I am certain that children are among your insureds. Therefore, having child psychologists on your panel would be a cost-effective means of addressing these children's mental health needs.

As a clinical child psychologist, I assess and treat children from birth through 17 years of age with a wide variety of complaints. My theoretical approach and training are in the behavioral and cognitive behavioral therapies, which are, of course, compatible with the managed care philosophy of brief, targeted intervention. I am also quite familiar with measuring outcomes in therapy and do this routinely in my practice.

You will see from my vita, which is attached, that I have 10 years of experience in clinical child psychology since becoming licensed. I understand that your provider panel is currently closed, but since this appears to be an unfilled need, I am requesting that you send me an application form. I will call you in 2 weeks to discuss the possibility of adding my name to your provider list, but feel free to call me with any additional questions you may have in the meanwhile.

Thank you for taking time to consider my request.

Sincerely,

Ima Helper, Ph.D.
1 Mental Place
Anytown, Anystate
(123) 555-4567
Enclosure

they do not seem particularly interested, it is important that the clinician request that the company send an application or other materials to facilitate the process, with the goal of the clinician being added to the panel of providers. The clinician will need to call again to follow up on the status of the application. If the response is "don't call us, we'll call you," the clinician can call anyway after a reasonable period of time (perhaps a month). Similarly, the clinician can find out when the review committee meets again and can call just after that meeting. If the representative refuses to send an application, it is appropriate to ask when the managed care organization anticipates their panel will be open again. Often when companies merge or are sold (a frequent occurrence in managed behavior health care), panels become reopened after an initial adjustment as it becomes apparent contracts cannot be fulfilled with existing panel members.

States have varying laws regarding provider applications, so clinicians should check with their state psychological association regarding any laws or regulations on access to provider panels. In some cases, the managed care company may be required to send an application if asked, and each state may have unique laws regarding that process. In Chapter 3, we discussed what the clinician can do if denied entry onto a panel.

ACCESSING PANELS AS A "SPECIALIST" OR "SUBSPECIALIST"

As more companies, clinicians, and patients realize the importance of specific, competent services, greater numbers of provider panels are being developed from those trained as specialists and subspecialists (depending on one's nomenclature and a company's benefit package), such as geropsychology, clinical child/pediatric psychology, forensic psychology, marriage/family counseling, and alcohol and substance abuse counseling. Each of these areas is developing its own identity and core training experiences. We believe that, if a clinician has specialty skills, this can make him or her more attractive to those better companies who are concerned with quality services, efficacy, efficiency, and enhanced consumer satisfaction. The field has advanced, in our view, sufficiently to justify the value of specialists. Thus, subspecialty skills, such as child and pediatric specialty training, can sometimes make a clinician more desirable to a managed care organization.

As we have emphasized, it is essential that clinicians do some research on the managed care organization and its served populations. Indeed, knowledge is strength, especially for the specialist. For example, knowing that the adult enrollees of a managed care company are primarily ages 20–45, then higher proportions of them are likely to be parents with typical concerns for their children. The clinician should also be familiar with types of mental health problems in the local community in order to identify niches of opportunity for specialty panels. One of us (MCR) lives in an area in which (for historical reasons of availability of services at one time—not causative) there exists a larger than average population of children who are deaf and their parents. The area also has a substantial group of children with autism. Although schools may provide educationally related services to these populations, ancillary mental health services may be required by the families who are covered by local and national employers' plans. Ability to provide services to these populations may have managed care organizations seeking out the clinician rather than the other way around.

Whatever the community/population needs are, the specialty requirements of these types of groups can be pointed out to the managed care company that has such enrollees if the clinician has done his or her homework. On the other hand, if an organization has just signed a contract to provide Medicare services to retirees, a *child* specialist is unlikely to be successful in applying to the newly created panels. Thus, knowing the types of services for which managed care contracts have been made (including or excluding children from the plans) can also increase a clinician's chances of gaining access to a panel based on specialty ability and training. The clinician can check the list of current providers to determine if any other specialists are included. If not, there may be an institutional bias against them or there may have been no previous specialists with such ability who have applied. The clinician will need to be more aggressive in overcoming these adverse circumstances by demonstrating the value of specialty panels for the marketing of managed care plans (not to mention the improved services for children, adolescents, and families).

The clinician might start a specialty application letter by briefly reviewing any local market information available, such as the need for mental health benefits for children, documenting the benefits of providing services that are appropriate to children and therefore not the same as those offered to adults, medical cost offsets gained by providing appropriate mental health services, and similar documentation supporting the clinician's case (see Chapter 7 for more information). This should be a brief, one- to two-paragraph introduction.

If the clinician has information on a particular managed care company's clients, he or she may be able to provide data on the number of children likely covered by their policies and, given the data on prevalence of mental health concerns in children, the estimated number of beneficiaries who are likely to need specialized services. If other child/pediatric psychologists are on the panel, the clinician may be able to use this information, possibly along with information on those other providers' wait times, to justify the need to add another specialist provider to the panel. The more specific information on how the clinician can aid the managed care company, the more seriously the company is likely to take an unsolicited application.

Next, the clinician can describe what he or she can offer that the managed care company does not currently provide. Although the clinician may also list services that are provided by others, it will help if there is a clear statement of the uniqueness of one's services or training. If the list of services offered is lengthy, an attachment can be used while providing a sentence or two summarizing those services in the body of the letter.

In applying to a panel as a specialist, the child clinician may wish to identify what he or she considers essential characteristics of the specialty. These specialty characteristics might include detailing:

- Academic courses in child and adolescent development, developmental psychopathology, child and family assessment techniques (as well as Continuing Education workshops taken since graduation)
- Specialized intervention strategies including child/adolescent therapy, parent interventions, family therapy, and school and community interventions, especially those brief interventions compatible with managed care parameters
- Supervised practicum experiences and clinical internship training directly related to interventions with children, adolescents, and their families (and specified treatment approaches, e.g., behavior therapy, parent–child interaction therapy)
- Postdoctoral fellowships in settings serving children
- Professional positions primarily serving populations of children and families (e.g., outpatient/inpatient treatment programs, comprehensive mental health centers, children's hospitals, consulting with group homes, etc.)

Of course, just listing these on a vita may not make them apparent or relevant to the panel representative. The clinician needs to make the case that these are extraordinary and useful to the managed care organization as compared to generalist training. The clinician might explain in a letter, by telephone, or in person how his or her particular background translates into the ability to serve children better and more cost-effectively. We also caution all clinicians not to overreach in claiming specialty credentials. The *Ethical Principles of Psychologists* (American Psychological Association, 1992) apply. The *Ethical Principles* state:

> Principle A: Competence. Psychologists strive to maintain high standards of competence in their work. They recognize the boundaries of their particular competencies and the limitations of their expertise. They provide only those services and use only those techniques for which they are qualified by education, training, or experience (p. 1599).

To claim unearned specialty credentials is not only unethical, but children/families, managed care payers, and the clinician all would be poorly served by such exaggerations.

Most states license psychologists generically (i.e., without reference to specialty in the title). However, many require a formal statement presented to the licensing authority in which core areas of competence are declared. In these cases, it behooves the clinician to have articulated a specialty with the licensure board to be able to demonstrate to the managed care organization that one's credentials are not created ad hoc to fit the reimbursement situation. Membership in one of the national organizations serving the child/pediatric field and one's attempts to remain current with the field through journals may demonstrate strong interests, although these are not credentials in and of themselves. Diplomate status in a speciality, such as confirmation by the American Board of Professional Psychology, may enhance one's marketability (e.g., in clinical psychology, health psychology, neuropsychology, or forensic psychology). In justifying a claim for specialty status, clinicians may want to become familiar with how the field nationally views specialty training. Practitioners claiming the titles of family psychologist, school psychologist, applied developmental psychologist, and clinical child psychologist, among others, often assert that special and specific training is required for a clinician to use such titles. However, it must be noted that *legal* requirements are applied by the state licensing board. A group of psychologists from a variety of specialty psychology groups (e.g., school, clinical child, pediatric, family) have outlined a model for training psychologists to provide services for children, adolescents, and their families. The following courses of study have been outlined as necessary components of training for this "generic specialty":

- Life span developmental psychology
- Life span developmental psychopathology
- Child, adolescent, and family assessment methods
- Intervention strategies

  □ Child/adolescent interventions
  □ Parent interventions
  □ Family interventions
  □ School and community interventions

- Research methods and systems evaluation
- Professional, ethical, and legal issues pertaining to children, adolescents, and families
- Issues of diversity
- The role of multiple disciplines and service delivery systems

- Prevention, family support, and health promotion
- Social issues affecting children, adolescents, and families
- Specialized applied experiences in assessment, intervention, and consultation (Roberts et al., submitted for publication).

The clinician wishing to access a provider panel as a specialist or subspecialist may wish to use this model as an outline for demonstrating a specialty background. The clinician should also be aware that a commission has been formed within the APA to formally recognize specialties and proficiencies. Child-related organizations and other interested groups are formulating petitions for recognition in areas of family, school, and clinical child psychology (in addition to others in clinical, health, and neuropsychology). Some of these petitions, as a side effect of formalization, may exclude some practicing clinicians who currently claim specialist status. This activity bears watching.

Finally, with regard to accessing panels as a child-oriented specialist, the clinician can utilize the information provided in Chapter 7 about the value of psychosocial interventions with children demonstrated by the professional literature. Additionally, when describing the value of a specialty background, the clinician can cite the position paper by Roberts and colleagues (submitted for publication), "A Model for Training Psychologists to Provide Services for Children and Adolescents: Competence to meet the mental health needs of children, adolescents, and their families is tied directly to training for that specialty competence" (p. 7). Furthermore, the complexity of child and family problems often requires an ability to work with a variety of settings, professionals, and contexts, such as medical/pediatric, community, and schools. Generalists are not likely to have as many of the necessary skills and competencies in working in these settings. The manner in which the child specialty clinician presents himself or herself, thus, may enhance the likelihood of becoming a panelist and getting listed as a specialist. Indeed, having highly qualified specialists on the managed care provider panel can be a strong selling point to potential buyers. This aspect can be pointed out to the managed care organization.

WRITING BEHAVIORAL AND MEASURABLE TREATMENT GOALS

Most managed care plans require that additional treatment beyond the first few sessions be precertified. In order to have treatment authorized, behavioral treatment goals are generally required. Unfortunately, the managed care companies have tended to have written guidelines for what is acceptable, but have been unwilling to share these with providers. In addition, these guidelines are most often written regarding adult patients and may be difficult to apply to children's services. Treatment goals must generally be measurable or quantifiable and must be written with the *child* as the target for change. In other words, "Mrs. Smith will give direct commands 50% of the time" would not be acceptable when Mrs. Smith is not the identified patient. The goal could be modified to "Jason will comply with adult commands 70% of the time," which may be more acceptable to the managed care organization.

Treatment goals generally fall into three categories: problem-oriented, goal-oriented, and process-oriented. A single treatment plan may include aspects of all three. Managed care organizations typically adopt the medical model of problem-oriented goals, or decreasing symptoms (Sikorszky, 1996).

As previously noted, identifying the patient's or parents' reasons for seeking therapy is an important initial step in developing a treatment plan. Behavioral treatment goals are generally targeted to a particular symptom or behavior, which is the target of treatment. If a child patient has trouble falling asleep because of anxiety and the goal is for her to go to sleep within a shorter period of time, the clinician might have her keep charts of (1) her anxiety level prior to falling asleep and (2) the amount of time she estimates it took to fall asleep each night (to be noted the following morning). This sort of documentation has several advantages: The child is involved in the treatment outcome process and can see his or her progress, especially if either the clinician or the child graphs the changes. Parents can see progress on covert problems they might otherwise not be able to accurately evaluate. Although not as formal as research-oriented outcome measures, the clinician can provide the managed care company with documentation that the treatment works. If treatment is not working, the clinician will have that information early enough to make changes and then measure outcomes again.

Each managed care organization requires different information in their unique format, although most include some similar characteristics. To be acceptable, a treatment plan generally must:

- Address the medical necessity of the diagnosis, condition, or problem and list goals and objectives that focus on the fastest and most efficient means of decreasing symptoms. Other problems are expected to be referred to self-help groups, schools, or other organizations.
- Emphasize short-term treatments that fit the managed care organization case manager's interpretation of level-of-care guidelines.
- Emphasize operationally defined behavioral outcomes that are solution-oriented.
- Focus primarily on cognitive-behavioral or behavioral interventions.
- Decrease reliance on formal psychological testing and seldom recommend it.

- Involve the therapist and patient working together, and include the patient's concerns, motivations, and culture.
- Include family, teachers, and other support systems; emphasize homework assignments; and spread out treatment sessions when therapy is about to end in order to increase the patient's independence from the clinician and help treatment gains generalize to other settings and become part of the patient's adaptive functioning.
- Include treatment outcome and customer satisfaction and other form of measures (unless the managed care organization does its own satisfaction measure) (Sikorszky, 1996). An example of a satisfaction measure is presented later in this chapter.

    Treatment planning often is dictated and/or mandated by external managed care entities and is disliked by many clinicians. In practice, treatment planning usually focuses on filling out forms in ways the clinician or treatment team guesses the managed care organization case manager will accept. Also, the treatment planning process often seems to be after-the-fact and disconnected from the clinical and therapeutic process. Clinicians rarely see it as adding to their therapeutic success and usually consider it another way that managed care has managed to waste their time (Giolas, 1996).

Hembree-Kigin and McNeil (1995) have developed a user-friendly (and seemingly managed care-friendly) book that contains a protocol for parent training for children with behavior problems. The treatment protocol is specific, yet flexible, and could be helpful with a variety of children who present with problem behaviors. This book also includes handouts for parents to take home, prescribed homework assignments, and pre- and posttreatment evaluation forms. It includes forms for the clinician to document improvements in the parents' skills as well as parent and teacher evaluation forms. In all of these ways, this treatment protocol appears to be managed care-friendly. In fact, Klett and Rashap (1996) are evaluating the use of this protocol within a managed care environment at the Rockville, Maryland satellite clinic of Children's National Medical Center. Silverman and Kurtines (1996) have a similar book on treatment of children's anxiety disorders that is quite easily understood and applied and that also contains sample forms. The push for manualized treatments for specific problems has increased the availability of such protocols to the practicing clinician, and more are expected to be available soon.

Despite the development of empirically based treatment protocols, some outcomes are more difficult to measure than others. It is often helpful for the clinician to identify the strategies proposed to produce a change and state the behavioral goals in those terms. For example, if the goal is to increase the

---

BOX 4.2. SAMPLE MANAGED CARE
TREATMENT REQUEST FORM

Managed Behavioral Healthcare Treatment Request Form

Patient Name: _____ Date of Birth: _____ Member/Sponsor #: _____
Address: _____ Health Plan Group: _____

Provider Name: _____ Address: _____ Phone: _____ Fax: _____
License type: _____ License #: _____ TIN# or SSAN: _____

Axis I: _____ Axis II: _____ Axis III: _____ Axis IV: _____ Axis V: _____

First date of service: _____ Last visit date: _____ Number of visits requested: _____
Do you anticipate requesting additional visits after this request? _____ Type of treatment: _____
Frequency of visits: _____ How long will this patient be in treatment? _____ weeks

Other services needed: ____ Psychological testing ____ Psychiatric referral ____ Psychotherapist ___No other services
Preferred provider: _____ Referral Reason: _____

Treatment plan:
1. Primary care provider: _____ Has provider been notified the patient is seeing you? _____
2. Medications (name, dose, prescribed by): _____

3. Clinical formulation of patient's problem: _____

4. Progress to date: _____

5. Problems in treatment, reason for requesting additional visits: _____

6. Criteria for treatment termination: _____

Problem list and treatments:
1. Primary problem, symptoms: _____ Proposed treatment: _____ Behavioral/measureable goal:
   _____   _____   _____

2. Second problem, symptoms: _____ Proposed treatment: _____ Behavioral/measureable goal:
   _____   _____   _____

3. Other problem, symptoms: _____ Proposed treatment: _____ Behavioral/measureable goal:
   _____   _____   _____

Treatment termination summary: (for patients completing treatment)
1. List goals met: _____
2. Were there any problems which remain unresolved? _____ If so, what do you recommend be done? _____

3. Have you made any referrals for the above problems (if so, to whom)? _____

Provider's signature: _____ Date: _____

---

self-esteem of Susan, a teenage patient, the clinician could use changes on a self-esteem scale as one measure or could state, "Susan will make 5 positive self-statement on 5 of 7 days," and then ask Susan to write down each time she makes a positive self-statement. It is not always necessary to retest children to document changes, but it is sometimes desirable, particularly if the test is not burdensome or overly expensive to administer. Behavioral checklists and self-report questionnaires are usually easy to administer and score and provide adequate documentation for these purposes. A sample request form for managed care approval of a treatment plan is presented in Box 4.2.

OUTCOME MEASUREMENT AND EVALUATION

Outcome evaluation in clinical practice is becoming increasingly important, with the demand from third-party payers for documentation of success. In addition, evaluation of one's business practices and their success is also important, and will be further discussed in Chapter 5. Accountability has become critically important for clinicians hoping to join or remain on managed care panels. Even though empirical evaluation of psychotherapy began in the 1950s, outcome measurement is still in a formative phase, with great variability among providers and payers in terms of what is offered, what is acceptable, and how to collect adequate information. Publication of a *Consumer Reports* article that reported survey evidence gathered retrospectively indicating that psychotherapy works and that more therapy is better started a renewed debate over outcome measurement in psychotherapy (Consumers Union, 1995). Kazdin (1996) argues that although validated treatments are generally a good idea, in clinical practice one must also be flexible in order to ensure that the treatment is tailored to the client and the range of problems presented, and to modify treatments that are not working. Clinicians must be certain that they apply validated treatments correctly, and that clients are compliant with the treatment proposed. In some cases, other important agents of change (teachers, parents) must also comply with treatment requirements. The evidence that therapy is helpful does not insure that any particular patient improves, improves sufficiently, or improves in all problem areas targeted. These issues are summarized in Chapter 7. In this section, we want to describe some ways the clinician can adapt to the managed care environment by measuring therapeutic outcomes in real practice.

An important issue to consider in outcome evaluation is what the individual's goal is versus what some other entity's goal may be (Strupp, 1996). Many people seek help for problems that do not fit traditional DSM-IV diagnostic criteria, concerns that we might classify as variations on normal development or concerns of daily living. Sometimes a goal for one person would be unacceptable for another. Although it has become the norm that managed care will only reimburse patients for disorders fitting within DSM-IV criteria, we must recognize that there are many other legitimate reasons for seeking psychotherapy. If the current trend for managed care to pay only for treatment of "diagnosable" conditions continues, then outcome measurement for "undiagnosable" conditions may be ignored since the clinician's income and job are not dependent on it.

Studies of outcome in mental health treatment are full of problems and often do not reflect the same process as that which occurs in real-life clinical settings. Pfeiffer and Shott (1996) recommend that outcome measurement should:

1	Include clinician assessment and self-assessment
2	Collect inpatient measures during hospitalization as well as follow up data postdischarge, and
3	Collect outcome measures at several points during therapy

Howard, Lueger, Maling, and Martinovich (1993) described a phase model of psychotherapy outcome and demonstrated that, in adults, improvement progresses through a series of predictable phases. This model argues against the cost-containment approach of using active, directive therapists engaging exclusively in time-limited, ultra-brief therapy. Howard et al. (1993) state that "Therapeutic interventions are likely to be most effective when they focus on changing phase-specific problems when those problems are most accessible to change" (p. 684).

Dr. Paul Clement (1996) proposed an extensive data collection system for both patient outcome/treatment success and for practice management data. Clement proposes more extensive assessment of outcome using instruments borrowed from the program evaluation literature. In particular, he recommends the use of Goal Attainment Scaling (Kiresuk & Sherman, 1968) combined with Global Assessment of Functioning (GAF) ratings to evaluate overall outcome as well as outcome on specified goals. Goal Attainment Scaling involves rating outcome on a five-point scale as follows: (−2) much worse than expected, (−1) worse than expected, (0) the most likely outcome, (+1) better than expected, and (+2) much better than expected. GAF ratings allow for finer discrimination of levels by using nine levels that are roughly equivalent to ten GAF points per level. The clinician and patient (or parent) jointly identify several goals for treatment outcome and specify functioning levels that are paired with a point level on the scale. The level of functioning at the initial visit is established and progress is monitored on an ongoing basis until, ideally, the patient (parent) and clinician agree that there is no need for further treatment. Multiple studies using this scale have been published, although it has not been widely used in private practice.

There are some significant problems with this method of outcome evaluation. Agreement among the various raters may be low or high. The psychometric properties of such lists may be weak and, therefore, less useful in research or in outcome evaluation over a broader scale. These may be most useful to a single patient and therapist dyad. Treatment effects are difficult to separate from a therapist goal-setting bias. Sometimes goals may be too easy or too difficult to attain, yet be included in the analysis. The actual setting of goals may be therapeutic and confounded with expectations for improvement. The concurrent validity of goal attainment is poorly correlated with other outcome measures. Numerous variations on the Goal Attainment Scaling exist, making it difficult to make comparisons from practitioner to practitioner. It is a very time-intensive procedure, especially initially, and is therefore potentially expensive to accomplish (Lambert & Brown, 1996). Box 4.3 illustrates how the GAF might be used in practice.

Because of some of these difficulties, other commentators proposed an alternative system for evaluating outcome that is somewhat more efficient in terms of time involvement. Lambert and Brown (1996) propose supplementing individualized goals with standardized clinical rating scales and using both to evaluate treatment outcome. This provides the advantage of comparison with a normative group, with other patients' pretest and/or posttest scores, or comparison of a patient against some accepted standard of improvement, where available. Such standardized scales can generally be used to evaluate clinical change in relation to a cutoff score, based on national norms, for improvement. For example, the Eyberg Child Behavior Inventory (Eyberg & Ross, 1978) reliably measures changes in child compliance from session to session and can be repeated as often as indicated. The Children's Depression Inventory (Kovacs, 1981) can be used repeatedly to measure changes in reported depressive symptoms.

In this type of outcome evaluation, the patient (parent) and clinician jointly develop measurable goals for change. Each session, it is recommended that the clinician and/or parent rate change from the previous session. In addition, the child (if old enough) completes a standard rating scale before the therapy session begins. In reality, many clinical child psychologists will not be able to follow these standard adult therapy outcome procedures because of age limitations and limited availability of standardized child outcome measures. However, when standardized scales are available, the progress on both individualized goals and standardized scales can be displayed graphically after data are entered into a computer or after hand calculations are made and placed on a graph. The reader who is interested in calculating clinically significant change on a particular instrument is referred to Jacobson, Follette, and Revenstorf (1986) for a review of the statistical methodology.

In addition to broad band assessment devices, several other narrow band scales are available for measuring specific characteristics. Other, more simplified and individualized systems, such as thermometer and happy face scales, are often used by pediatric and child clinical psychologists in private practice (see Box 4.4). Children's ratings on such scales can be translated into numerical form and statistically analyzed. Advantages of frequent outcome measurement include demonstrable progress to patients and managed care companies; when progress is not seen, the treatment plan can be modified accordingly.

Wholesale purchasers of health care services are demanding that measurement of clinical outcomes be incorporated in the health care delivery system and that treatment decisions be based on sound empirical evidence for efficacy and value rather than just on cost savings or other financial considerations. In response

BOX 4.3 GAF/GAS-TYPE RATING SCALE FOR MEASURING TREATMENT OUTCOME FOR SCHOOL AVOIDANCE

Level of functioning	Score	Description of each level	Date of evaluation
Good functioning	9	I get up and get ready for school, and arrive on time 5 days per week. I do not argue with or complain to my parents about going to school or about how much I dislike school. I remember to take all my books and homework and to turn in my completed homework.	
Slight problem	8	I get up and get to school on time 5 days per week. On 1 or 2 days/week I argue with or complain to my parents about going to school, but I go anyway without being late. All the above statements are true except for that.	12/12/96
Some problem	7	I get up and get to school on time 5 days/week. On most days (3–4/week), I argue with or complain to my parents about school. All the above statements are true except for that.	
Moderate difficulty	6	I get up and get to school on time 4–5 days per week. Every day I argue with or complain to my parents about school, and my mom sometimes has to pull me out of bed (1–2 times/week). I take my books and homework, but my teacher has to ask me for my homework 1–2 days/week.	11/6/96

BOX 4.3. (*Continued*)

Serious problem	5	I stayed home from school saying I was sick when I really wasn't 1–2 days in the past month. All of the above statements are true except for that.	
Major impairment	4	All of the above is true except that I stayed home from school 3–4 days in the past month when I was not really sick.	10/8/96
Inability to function	3	The statements in the preceding level are true except I stayed home from school 5 or more days in the past month when I was not truly sick.	
Some danger of hurting self or others	2	Not applicable.	

Adapted from Clement, 1996.

---

to this demand, the major managed care companies are moving to develop the methodology to incorporate measurement of clinical outcomes into their delivery systems. The current generation of information systems is referred to as Clinical Information Systems (Sikorszky, 1996). Managed care companies are developing practice management software that will include the collection of clinical data through the use of electronic patient records or scannable forms that can be mailed or faxed to the managed care company. A well-designed electronic patient record can incorporate both ideographic data including individualized treatment plans and goals and standardized measures of patient functioning and improvement (Todd, Jacobus, & Boland, 1992). Managed care companies will then be able to profile providers based on clinical outcomes obtained and the cost of obtaining those outcomes. To do this, standardized outcome measures that can be compared across a broad sample of providers and patients will be required. Child mental health data will not likely be included in the evaluation measures initially proposed. Therefore, child-oriented clinicians have the opportunity to develop suitable instruments and procedures to introduce to managed care entities.

BOX 4.4 EXAMPLES OF NON-VERBAL OUTCOME SCALES OR USE WITH CHILDREN

1. Thermometer scale (example; use with anxious child)

—4 Very, very anxious   Instructions to child: "Rate how
—3 Pretty anxious   anxious you felt when _____.
—2 A little anxious   (The clinician defines when the
—1 Just a bit anxious   anxiety ratings should be taken
—0 Not at all anxious   and what should be measured,
                         with input from the child and
                         parents.)

2. Happy face scale (example; use with depressed child)

Great, terrific	Pretty good	Neither good nor bad	Pretty bad	Terrible, awful

      1   2   3   4   5

"Which face tells how you felt when _____?"

NOTE: The wording on these scales can be changed to match the feeling being measured. For example, the thermometer could be used to measure "worried," "pain," or "sad" instead of anxious if that is the feeling being measured.

The following five steps have been recommended for selecting an outcome measure:

1   Decide what to measure (formalize treatment goals with behavioral objectives for each component).
2   Determine if unintended side effects need to be measured (either positive or negative).
3   Organize a plan for assessment.
4   Determine which outcome measures are applicable to the situation.
5   Determine rules for selecting specific assessment instruments (the following questions might guide selection):

□ Is it practical (including administration time and scoring ease)?
□ Is it relevant to the target group (high reliability and validity)?

☐ Does it use behavioral descriptions?

☐ Does it use multiple informants, including parents and teachers?

☐ What are the psychometric properties, including reliability, validity, and sensitivity to change?

☐ What is the cost to purchase and administer, store information, score, use the results, and possible expense due to errors or complications?

☐ How easy will it be for nonprofessionals to understand?

☐ Is it compatible with professional standards of practice?

☐ Is it useful in real-world applications? (Pfeiffer & Shott, 1996, p. II.E.5).

The Youth Outcome Questionnaire (Y-OQ) (Wells, Burlingame, Lambert, Hoag, & Hope, 1996) is a recently developed outcome measure for children 4–17 years old that addresses the needs of both clinicians and managed care administrators. The Y-OQ and its adult counterpart, the Outcome Questionnaire, or OQ-45, were developed with four main objectives. They were instruments that would be: (1) used each therapy session to monitor outcomes and progress, (2) quick to administer, (3) able to detect change over brief time periods, and (4) inexpensive to purchase. The Y-OQ was developed from a variety of source material, including review of child clinical treatment reports, focus groups of consumers (including children, adolescents, and their parents) who had received mental health treatment in a managed care organization, focus groups with various mental health providers, and review of treatment charts to identify treatment-related changes associated with stated therapeutic goals. From these sources, six content areas or subscales were developed: Intrapersonal Distress, Somatic, Interpersonal Relations, Critical Items, Social Problems, and Behavioral Dysfunction. These six domains cover the majority of problems presented to child clinicians, with the exception of developmental and academic problems. The first page of the Y-OQ is reprinted in Box 4.5.

The test developers also recognized that there are mitigating factors that may impact treatment outcome with children and adolescents. The Y-OQ PA is a separate, ten-item prognostic assessment questionnaire that addresses most potential mitigating factors for success. The psychometric properties of the Y-OQ, based on a sample of children 6–17 years old, are acceptable. The total score is the one typically used to track change. Average classification accuracy (inpatient, outpatient, community normal) is 85%, with inpatient the most accurate prediction (90.5%). The Y-OQ is highly correlated (.84) with the Total Problem Score on the Child Behavior Checklist. Wells et al. (1996) describe how this instrument can be used by clinicians to develop treatment plans and track patient progress and by a managed care organization to report treatment effec-

BOX 4.5. FIRST PAGE OF THE YOUTH OUTCOME QUESTIONNAIRE (Y-OQ 2.0). REPRINTED WITH PERMISSION OF QUESTIONNAIRE AUTHORS AND THE AMERICAN PROFESSIONAL CREDENTIALING SERVICES, P.O. BOX 346, STEVENSON, MARYLAND 21153

Youth Outcome Questionnaire (Y-OQ™2.0)

Child's Name _____ ID# _____ Today's Date _____

Child's Date of Birth _____ Child's Sex: Male ___ Female ___ Parent/Guardian _____

PURPOSE: The Y-OQ™2.0 is designed to describe a wide range of troublesome situations, behaviors, and moods that are common in children and adolescents. You may discover that some of the items do not apply to your child's current situation. If so, please do not leave these items blank, but check the "Never or almost never" category. When you begin to complete the Y-OQ™2.0 you will see that you can easily make your child look as healthy or unhealthy as you wish. Please do not do that. If you are as accurate as possible it is more likely that you will be able to receive the help that you are seeking for your child.

DIRECTIONS:
- Read each statement carefully.
- Check the box that most accurately describes your child during the past week.
- Decide how true this statement is for your child during the past 7 days.
- Check only one answer for each statement and erase unwanted marks clearly.

EXAMINATION COPY

PLEASE COMPLETE BOTH SIDES

My Child:	Never or Almost Never	Rarely	Sometimes	Frequently	Almost Always or Always
1. Wants to be alone more than other children of the same age	☐	☐	☐	☐	☐
2. Complains of dizziness or headaches	☐	☐	☐	☐	☐
3. Doesn't participate in activities that were previously enjoyable	☐	☐	☐	☐	☐
4. Argues or is verbally disrespectful	☐	☐	☐	☐	☐
5. Is more fearful than other children of the same age	☐	☐	☐	☐	☐
6. Cuts school or is truant	☐	☐	☐	☐	☐
7. Cooperates with rules and expectations	☐	☐	☐	☐	☐
8. Has difficulty completing assignments, or completes them carelessly	☐	☐	☐	☐	☐
9. Complains or whines about things being unfair	☐	☐	☐	☐	☐
10. Experiences trouble with her/his bowels, such as constipation or diarrhea	☐	☐	☐	☐	☐
11. Gets into physical fights with peers or family members	☐	☐	☐	☐	☐
12. Worries and can't get certain ideas off his/her mind	☐	☐	☐	☐	☐
13. Steals or lies	☐	☐	☐	☐	☐
14. Is fidgety, restless, or hyperactive	☐	☐	☐	☐	☐
15. Seems anxious or nervous	☐	☐	☐	☐	☐
16. Communicates in a pleasant and appropriate manner	☐	☐	☐	☐	☐
17. Seems tense, easily startled	☐	☐	☐	☐	☐
18. Soils or wets self	☐	☐	☐	☐	☐
19. Is aggressive toward adults	☐	☐	☐	☐	☐
20. Sees, hears, or believes things that are not real	☐	☐	☐	☐	☐
21. Has participated in self-harm (e.g. cutting or scratching self, attempting suicide)	☐	☐	☐	☐	☐
22. Uses alcohol or drugs	☐	☐	☐	☐	☐
23. Seems unable to get organized	☐	☐	☐	☐	☐
24. Enjoys relationships with family and friends	☐	☐	☐	☐	☐
25. Appears sad or unhappy	☐	☐	☐	☐	☐
26. Experiences pain or weakness in muscles or joints	☐	☐	☐	☐	☐
27. Has a negative, distrustful attitude toward friends, family members, or other adults	☐	☐	☐	☐	☐
28. Believes that others are trying to hurt him/her even when they are not	☐	☐	☐	☐	☐
29. Threatens to, or has run away from home	☐	☐	☐	☐	☐
30. Experiences rapidly changing and strong emotions	☐	☐	☐	☐	☐

SUBTOTALS

tiveness data to subscribers and to set empirically determined "appropriate" session limits via expectancy tables. These authors have also developed a screening version, the Y-OQ-11, to be used in a primary care setting in order to identify patients who might benefit from a referral for further psychological evaluation. They suggest that by screening patients in a fully capitated total health care system and initiating appropriate mental health services early on, total costs could be reduced. It would also seem that the Y-OQ-11 could be used to determine likely referral patterns for mental health professionals considering accepting capitated contracts.

CONSUMER SATISFACTION

In Chapter 7, we examine some of the empirical findings from consumer satisfaction research. In this section we will discuss some ways for the clinician to collect consumer satisfaction information, both to determine how one is doing and to present to managed care organizations one piece of information about outcomes.

Measures of satisfaction with psychological services are a useful way for clinicians to demonstrate the value of clinical interventions. Satisfaction ratings are typically taken during or after evaluation and treatment from several sources, including the child client, the parent or guardian, the source of the referral, and other consumers (e.g., school teachers). Increasingly, managed care companies are requiring clinicians to obtain satisfaction ratings either of their own devising or using a form provided by the company.

In fact, managed care companies themselves are conducting periodic evaluations of their own procedures and services by surveying those enrolled in a network. These often are in the form of consumer satisfaction questionnaires. Favorable ratings are trumpeted in advertising and sales pitches to employers who might contract with the company. Conceivably, the clinician as an individual practitioner or in a group/clinic could use the same type of data for demonstration of success to the company managers.

One behavioral health service provider distributed a letter to "colleagues" describing an 18-month customer satisfaction survey of patients and families. The letter reported:

> The overall satisfaction rate for 1994 was 95%. In response to the questions, "Would you recommend the center to a friend?, Did the services help? and Would you return to the center?," 92% responded positively. Of ten functions measured (Admissions, Finance, Discharge, Nursing, Psychiatry, Primary Therapist, Treatment Staff,

Treatment Schedule, Treatment Activity and Environment), good to excellent ratings rose from 79% to 92% during 1994. First quarter 1995 results indicate even greater improvement in patient and family satisfaction. With survey results from 81% of patients discharged, 96% reported overall satisfaction and responded positively that they would recommend our program to a friend or family member in need....We recently commissioned a random survey of referral sources throughout the metropolitan area regarding their perceptions of mental health care and specifically of The Kansas Institute. Thirty-one (31) were randomly selected from among those who had used our services in the previous 12 months. Of those, *100%* reported satisfaction with the services their referred patients had received! (Kearney, 1995)

Other companies have similarly advertised their own consumer satisfaction findings. Although the clinician personally could conduct the surveys, contracting with an independent agency or university program might enhance credibility. Such an arrangement might provide statistical and design expertise to improve the pay-off of information. As detailed in Chapter 7, there are a number of published examples of how satisfaction with services ratings can be obtained. The clinician might point to these data as further demonstration of the quality of care and value provided via psychological services. Many clinicians and clinical service programs regularly request feedback from the parents who were seen for their children's problems (e.g., in parenting training interventions) or whose children participated in therapy (see Box 4.6 for an example). In addition to parent satisfaction, clinicians may choose to assess satisfaction about service from those who referred patients (e.g., pediatricians) or who may have been called upon to implement treatment strategies (e.g., school teachers; see Box 4.7 for an example). Finally, ratings of satisfaction with services may be obtained from the children and adolescents served. Examples of clinical practices utilizing these types of satisfaction measures and examples of their data results are provided in Chapter 7.

The important factors in these types of consumer satisfaction surveys include ratings by parents, referring professionals (e.g., physicians, school personnel), and sometimes the child clients themselves. Ratings can be obtained, depending on the needs of the clinician, on the following factors:

- Overall satisfaction with services
- Perceptions of benefit, utility, or effectiveness of psychological evaluation and treatment

BOX 4.6. PARENT/CONSUMER SATISFACTION QUESTIONNAIRE

This questionnaire is part of our ongoing attempts to provide the very best treatment we can for you and your child. The feedback you give us will help us to evaluate and improve our services in the future. We are interested in your opinions, whether or not they are positive. Your help is appreciated. Please insert the completed form in the enclosed stamped envelop and mail it to the Clinic.

Please check the line indicating your response.

Overall, how satisfied are you with the services you received from the Clinic?

____1 very satisfied
____2 satisfied
____3 neutral
____4 dissatisfied
____5 very dissatisfied

The problems for which you were seeking treatment at the Clinic are at this time:

____1 greatly improved
____2 improved
____3 about the same
____4 worse
____5 considerably worse

The therapist's assistance and recommendations were:

____5 not helpful at all
____4 somewhat helpful
____3 neutral
____2 helpful
____1 very helpful

To what extent did our Clinic meet your needs?

____1 almost all were met
____2 most were met
____3 some were met
____4 not many were met
____5 none were met

I liked the following the best about the Clinic:

_____
_____
_____

(continued)

BOX 4.6. (*Continued*)

I would like to have the Clinic change the following:

_____

_____

_____

I would recommend the Clinic to a friend or relative:

    ____1 strongly recommend
    ____2 recommend
    ____3 neutral
    ____4 not recommend
    ____5 strongly not recommend

I found the therapist's assistance to be:

    ____1 excellent
    ____2 good
    ____3 neutral
    ____4 poor
    ____5 very poor

I found the staff to be:

    ____5 not helpful at all
    ____4 somewhat helpful
    ____3 neutral
    ____2 helpful
    ____1 very helpful

My overall rating of your Clinic is:

    ____5 very poor
    ____4 poor
    ____3 neutral
    ____2 good
    ____1 excellent

_____

Signature (optional)

(You do not need to sign this form unless you want to. However, being able to match your responses to the Clinic procedures would help us to determine how to improve them.)

(This questionnaire is based on items and concepts contained in Krahn, Eisert, & Fifield, 1990; Schroeder & Gordon, 1991; Forehand & McMahon, 1981.)

BOX 4.7. REFERRAL SOURCE SATISFACTION QUESTIONNAIRE

Dear doctor, school teacher, etc.

___(name of child)___ was referred to the Clinic by you on _____ .
We have now completed a number of sessions of psychological therapy.
The Clinic would appreciate your feedback regarding our services for this
child. This brief questionnaire is part of our ongoing attempts to provide
the very best treatment for referrals you make to the Clinic. The feedback
you give us will help us to evaluate and improve our services in the future.
We are interested in your opinions, whether or not they are positive. Your
help is appreciated. Please insert the completed form in the enclosed
stamped envelope and mail it to the Clinic.

Please check the line indicating your response.

Overall, how satisfied are you with the psychological services this child
received from the Clinic?

____1 very satisfied
____2 satisfied
____3 neutral
____4 dissatisfied
____5 very dissatisfied
____ Do not know

The problems for which you referred the child for treatment at the Clinic
are at this time:

____1 greatly improved
____2 improved
____3 about the same
____4 worse
____5 considerably worse
____ Do not know

The parents and/or child have reported that the therapist's assistance and
recommendations were:

____5 not helpful at all
____4 somewhat helpful
____3 neutral
____2 helpful
____1 very helpful
____ Do not know

To what extent did our Clinic meet the needs of the child and parent(s)?

____1 almost all were met

(continued)

BOX 4.7. (*Continued*)

_____2 most were met
_____3 some were met
_____4 not many were met
_____5 none were met
_____ Do not know

I found the oral feedback (telephone call/in person consultation) from the therapist (Clinic) to be:

_____1 excellent
_____2 good
_____3 neutral
_____4 poor
_____5 very poor
_____ Did not receive oral feedback

I found the written feedback (chart or report) from the therapist (Clinic) to be:

_____5 very poor
_____4 poor
_____3 neutral
_____2 good
_____1 excellent
_____ Did not receive written feedback

I found the response time between referral and follow-up to be:

_____1 excellent
_____2 good
_____3 neutral
_____4 poor
_____5 very poor
_____Cannot determine

I found the effectiveness of the intervention to be:

_____5 not helpful at all
_____4 somewhat helpful
_____3 neutral
_____2 helpful
_____1 very helpful
_____Do not know

I would refer other children and families to the Clinic:

_____1 strongly recommend
_____2 recommend
_____3 neutral

BOX 4.7. (*Continued*)

___4 not recommend
___5 strongly not recommend

My overall rating of your Clinic is:

___5 very poor
___4 poor
___3 neutral
___2 good
___1 excellent

(This questionnaire is based on items and concepts contained in Olson, Holden, Friedman, Faust, Kenning, & Mason, 1988; Rodrigue et al., 1995.)

- Perceptions of overall psychological/behavioral improvement (including improvements in specific behaviors or situations as dictated by the presenting problems, e.g., teasing/aggressiveness, social skills, self-concept, eating)
- Perceptions of meeting needs of presenting problems
- Ease and understandability of implementation of recommendations and therapeutic work
- Confidence in the clinician and his or her recommendations
- Perceptions of appropriateness of treatment approach taken by the clinician
- Predictions that the respondent would refer or recommend somebody else to the clinician
- Predictions that the respondent would return for assistance on other problems in the future
- Ratings of particular aspects of the program or clinic
- Specific advice given or recommendations
- Professional staff other than the clinician
- Office procedures
- Waiting area decor
- Response times to make appointment or return calls
- Questions for narrative answers for perceptions of the positive and negative aspects of the clinical services (e.g., What did you like most about services? What did you like least about services? What could be changed to improve services?)

■ Ratings from other professionals making referrals to the clinician: response time to acknowledging referral and providing feedback; quality of feedback whether oral or written; follow-up services; prediction of making future referrals to the clinician

Obtaining this information should not be approached just for purposes of public relations or gaining access to a managed care panel. Such information, if carefully collected and conceptualized, can assist the clinician in evaluating and improving various aspects of the practice. Value or perceived value is an important factor in marketing when there are several competing clinicians or groups in a practice. Periodic and repeated measures of satisfaction can outline for the clinician where improvements have been successful or further modification is needed. We think a critical point, however, is that the clinician is gathering data on his or her own practice. Having this information available and having the attitude that such evaluation is beneficial can convey the clinician's professionalism perhaps more than any signed assurance statement.

CLINICAL PROBLEMS NOT COVERED BY MANAGED CARE PLANS

The clinician may find it helpful to keep in mind that some legitimate goals for change are not covered by a family's health insurance policy. For example, a child may not have a diagnosable mental disorder, but the child and family may benefit from brief therapy for a problem behavior or situation. If that is the case, it will be necessary for the clinician to discuss with the parents the fact that a proposed treatment will not likely be covered by their insurance, but that the clinician feels the treatment is necessary and reasonable. The clinician can then discuss how they can expect to benefit from treatment and how long the treatment would take and at what cost, helping the family determine whether they are able and willing to pursue the treatment proposed.

In Chapter 3, we discussed the clinician's duty to discuss coverage issues, outline the legalities involved, and provide some examples of how patients can become informed about their policies (see particularly Box 3.1). The clinician can help the parents understand the value and comparative cost of mental health services in familiar terms when self-paying (e.g., "The evaluation will cost less than that new set of tires you just bought," "I know you have been planning to buy a big screen TV, but the cost of an evaluation and treatment for Johnny's school problems will be less than that and will go a long way toward helping him succeed"). If a clinician believes treatment will need to go on longer than anticipated, he or she can review the progress made and discuss whether the parents want to continue or are satisfied with the progress to date. If a clinician

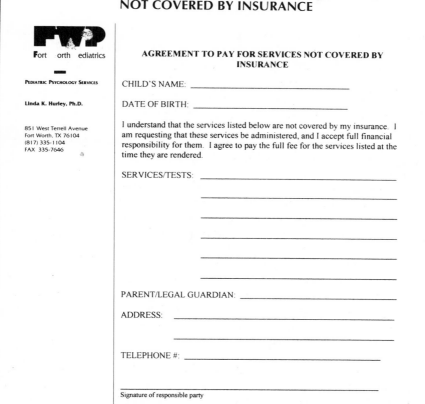

BOX 4.8. AGREEMENT TO PAY FOR SERVICES NOT COVERED BY INSURANCE

Fort **orth** **ediatrics**

PEDIATRIC PSYCHOLOGY SERVICES

Linda K. Hurley, Ph.D.

851 West Terrell Avenue
Fort Worth, TX 76104
(817) 335-1104
FAX 335-7646

AGREEMENT TO PAY FOR SERVICES NOT COVERED BY INSURANCE

CHILD'S NAME: _____

DATE OF BIRTH: _____

I understand that the services listed below are not covered by my insurance. I am requesting that these services be administered, and I accept full financial responsibility for them. I agree to pay the full fee for the services listed at the time they are rendered.

SERVICES/TESTS: _____

_____

_____

_____

_____

_____

PARENT/LEGAL GUARDIAN: _____

ADDRESS: _____

_____

TELEPHONE #: _____

_____
Signature of responsible party

_____
Printed name

_____
Billing address (if different from above)

_____

has been seeing a patient under an HMO's benefit plan and changes to fee-for-service, it is wise to ask the responsible party to sign an agreement to pay out-of-pocket with an understanding that their insurance plan will not covered the proposed services. This is sometimes required by provider managed care contracts. See Box 4.8 for an example of this type of form.

PRIORITIZE PROBLEMS, PRIORITIZE TREATMENTS

Managed care benefits are often designed for very brief treatment of specific problems, which sometimes means simply crisis management. However, children and families present with a wide range of complex problems. If a clinician is working within a managed care arrangement, he or she will be required to prioritize the problems presented. Even if the patient is fee-for-service, it is still a good idea to prioritize with the family what the joint treatment goals and acceptable outcomes are. This process is also helpful in identifying unrealistic goals ("Billy will never get angry") and helping the parents or child to accept a more reasonable goal ("when Billy gets angry, he will not hit his mother").

In some cases, families may present with a long list of important and legitimate needs, only some of which will be covered by their managed care plan. In this case, it is important for the clinician to review with the family what their insurance benefits cover and what things will not be covered. Families may have to make difficult choices in order to stay within their benefits plan (either family therapy or individual therapy for a daughter with anorexia, but not both). If the clinician feels both are necessary, he or she should provide the family with an honest opinion. The clinician can also help the family to choose between difficult alternatives, if necessary. In some cases, a family may decide to use their benefit plan for part of the needed treatments and pay out-of-pocket for others. By prioritizing problems and treatments, the clinician can help them make informed choices.

In other cases, lower priority problems may be put off for treatment at a later date. Most insurance plans "recycle" at the end of the benefit year, and, unless the family has totally used up their lifetime benefit, they may choose to work on the more pressing problem during the current benefit year. They can then return for help with other problems during their next benefit year. This prioritization also applies to families paying out-of-pocket: Their budget may not allow for extended treatment for all the problems, but they may be willing to meet with a clinician for a few sessions now and return for additional help later in the year. Targeting the most serious or stressful problem first can help get them back to a higher level of functioning and could help the clinician's reputation with the family as a reliable source of help.

Managed care companies generally seem to prefer drug treatments to psychotherapy since the cost to them is less, even though the long-term benefit is also less. If a clinician believes a child would benefit from therapy, the reasons should be discussed with the parents to help them understand their options as well as the benefits of the various choices. The clinician should not let a managed care plan dictate what he or she thinks is best, even if the reimbursement plan seems to be a family's only option.

USING TIME-LIMITED THERAPY

Managed care decision-making protocols put limits on the number of reimbursed sessions for each diagnosis as a cost-containment strategy. It is not apparent that these limits are based on any findings of how long therapy needs to be to gain a positive outcome. Nonetheless, these session limits have forced the mental health professions to utilize more time-limited modalities. This forced movement has often meant a shift to behaviorally based interventions for children and adolescents. Therapy for personal growth and personality change are generally not covered by managed care plans, as they tend to take longer than targeted behavioral treatments and have less proven value to managed care organizations. Of course, the lack of reimbursement through a managed care plan does not mean that a clinician cannot provide such treatment when requested; it means only that insurance will not likely cover it. Many families want treatment for a specific problem or behavior, even if they are not able to articulate that specific problem without some guidance and targeted questioning.

Insurance plans that include mental health benefits will often require the clinician to specify the number of visits anticipated for treatment of the specific problem. It is, therefore, a good idea to collect data on one's own practice patterns, including average number of visits for specific problems or diagnoses, even if standardized outcome measures are not used. (This idea is discussed further in Chapter 7.) Companies do keep data on utilization, and if a clinician tends to see patients for more sessions than other providers, he or she may be dropped from certain panels, or referrals will not be received from a managed care company for that reason. Many problems of childhood have well-documented behavioral treatments that tend to produce reliable behavior change in a reasonable amount of time. In many cases, use of these treatments will require increased involvement of parents, teachers, and other agents of change. When working with well-functioning and motivated families, these treatments can work well. However, with families that are illiterate, unmotivated, or overwhelmed with other stresses, change may be more difficult. The family's basic needs may be so overwhelming that they have little energy and few resources left for intensive treatment demands. In such cases, it may be more effective (and efficient) to provide more hands-on instruction and direct feedback such as illustrated by the parent–child interaction therapy (PCIT) protocol (Hembree-Kigin & McNeil, 1995). While this type of treatment will require more time from the clinician and will therefore be more expensive, we believe the clinician must tailor the treatment approach to the client's needs and abilities.

Unfortunately, managed care plans do not usually consider a family's circumstances when authorizing treatment or evaluating a clinician's ability to produce desired outcomes within a brief period of time. As Medicaid moves into a managed care model, these issues may become even more salient.

Bibliotherapy and Protocols

Over time, managed care organizations have embraced the concepts of using more treatment protocols and demanding more individual patient/parent responsibility for implementing change outside of therapy sessions. These concepts are often fulfilled by what have been called bibliotherapy and treatment protocols. These tools have existed in the clinicians' armamentarium for years (e.g., Roberts & Wright, 1982) with varying degrees of empirical support for their utility. Regardless, the clinician will find them useful for routinizing some interventions, assisting patients in making changes without extensive clinician contact, and publicizing one's practice. Before providing written materials for parents or others to read, it is necessary to be certain that the parents can read and do not object to reading. A surprising number of parents either do not read well or do not like to read, resulting in handouts being tossed in the trash as soon as they arrive home. With families who enjoy reading, bibliotherapy can be a very useful adjunct to face-to-face therapy and can speed the process of therapy. Providing families with books and other reading materials that describe behavioral or parenting techniques in detail can often speed the course of treatment. It is useful to send materials home to be read and then discuss them at the following visit, after parents have had a chance to identify their questions and possible problems in implementing changes.

Treatment protocols can also be sent home or to school with instructions on how to implement them and instructions to call the psychologist if questions arise. It is generally more successful to have at least a follow-up visit or two after giving handouts in order to troubleshoot and to plan for future fading of the treatment, if appropriate. If treatment protocols are given to parents to be implemented at home, it is generally necessary to review, step-by-step, what is actually expected. In order to cover each contingency, a protocol would need to be book-length, so discussing probable pitfalls with the parents is quite helpful in identifying the problems their particular child will likely present. Helping the parents anticipate where the protocol will break down and having a specific plan for how to respond will result in a more successful outcome. If the clinician simply sends the written treatment plan home without this discussion, parents will likely modify it to suit their needs, and the protocol will not be as likely to work. By anticipating problems and developing a contingency plan, the clinician helps the parents to develop a treatment approach that is really suited to their child. This will also likely increase their satisfaction and their likelihood of returning with future problems.

Box 4.9 presents a protocol or treatment plan used with a child with a feeding disorder. Although parts of the protocol are standard, it was developed to meet the needs of a particular child after the clinician completed an extensive interview with the parents, observed a family meal, and reviewed diet records and other assessment instruments. After the protocol had been written and tailored to meet the child's needs, the parents met with the psychologist to discuss potential problems and make minor modifications to the protocol. As of this writing, the parents have followed the protocol for 10 weeks and several additional modifications have been made to suit their specific circumstances (e.g., dining room arrangements). The managed care organization agreed to pay for treatment (but curiously has categorized it under "rehabilitation therapy"). However, payment had not been received for three months after the last visit. Outcome data (measured as number of bites eaten, plus ounces of milk, juice, or water consumed) indicated the child was improving. The managed care plan had not requested a copy of the treatment protocol or the outcome measures (and the clinician was not a network provider). However, these materials are available should they ever be needed. The family was seen for a total of five visits over a 13-week period, with telephone and/or mail check in every other week.

Homework

Whether they are labeled as such or not, most behavioral child interventions include the use of homework assignments for the child, the parents, or both. Such assignments are very compatible with managed care priorities. Homework assignments can help a child carry over the effect of treatment from one session to the next and can help keep parents informed of what their child is doing in therapy. Homework assignments for parents can also be helpful in making changes in behaviors that occur primarily outside of the therapy session, such as enuresis or school refusal. For example, the clinician can assign child homework when working with depressed adolescents (Wilkes, Belsher, Rush, & Frank, 1994). Additionally, clinicians frequently assign homework to parents of noncompliant children (Forehand & McMahon, 1981; Hembree-Kigin & McNeil, 1995). In fact, the majority of cognitive-behavioral therapy protocols include some homework at least part of the time. When homework is given, the clinician should usually write down step-by-step instructions for a younger child. Teenagers can be responsible for writing down their own homework assignments in many cases. Collecting data on behavioral assignments is a good use of homework ("keep a record of each time you practiced

BOX 4.9. FEEDING TREATMENT PLAN

Fort Worth Pediatrics

PEDIATRIC PSYCHOLOGY SERVICES

Linda K. Hurley, Ph.D.

851 West Terrell Avenue
Fort Worth, TX 76104
(817) 335-1104
FAX 335-7646

FEEDING TREATMENT PLAN

Name:
DOB:
Date of Plan:

1. All meals should be offered at the table or a kitchen counter. Do not allow your child to eat while roaming the house, or to get down from a meal and then return for additional bites of food. Try to feed your child separately from parents so you can fully attend to him during this treatment program. After he begins to eat better, he can join you for meals.

2. Set a timer for 25 minutes when you are ready for the meal to start. When the timer rings, the meal is over, even if your child is still eating. This will help insure that his behavior does not signal the end of the meal. When the timer rings, all of your child's foods and drinks should be removed and he should leave the table.

3. Schedule 3 meals and 2-3 snacks per day. Feed your child at these regular intervals. Meal and snack times should not vary more than 20 minutes either way. This will help your child learn to be hungry at certain times.

4. Do not offer any drinks or food for 30 minutes prior to a meal or 20 minutes before a snack. Drinking liquids or eating small snacks will decrease hunger for the meal. Do not allow your child to begin a meal with a drink. Offer *one sip* of a drink (e.g., milk) after he has eaten a bite of food. If you have trouble controlling the amount he takes from the cup, pour only a small sip into the cup and then give it to him.

5. Food quantity hierarchy:
    Step 1 - Your child must eat one bite (at least 1/8 teaspoon) of a preferred food before having a drink of milk. Once he has eaten a bite of food, he may have *one small sip* of milk. Note: if he takes several bites of food before drinking, he may have a larger drink of milk, but not more than 2 oz. at a time.
    Step 2 - Your child must eat one bite of a non-preferred food, then one bite of a preferred food before having a drink. After he has eaten the two bites, he may have a small sip of milk.
    Step 3 - Your child must eat one bite (1/4 teaspoon) of a non-preferred food and two bites (1/4 teaspoon each) of preferred food(s) before taking a sip of milk.
    Step 4 - Follow above directions, but he must eat 2 bites of non-preferred foods, then a sip of milk if desired, then 4 bites of preferred foods, then another sip of milk.
    Step 5 - Continue to increase the amount of food required between drinks.

BOX 4.9. (*Continued*)

Write down what step you are on and how your child did. Bring the record to your next appointment so we can see how he is progressing. Also write down what and how much food you offer as well as how much he actually consumes.

Start out each meal with the above hierarchy. Allow your child to finger-feed or use a utensil, as he prefers. If he does not take a bite within 60 seconds, place the food on a spoon and offer it to him (either so he can feed himself, or you feed him).

6. When your child succeeds, praise and attend to him. Overdo your praise and attention to him while he is eating well. If needed, you may verbally prompt ("take a bite," "swallow") once every 60-90 seconds, but not any more often. If you prompt more often, you are paying attention to the behavior you want to eliminate (not eating). Be sure that you avoid talking to him or interacting with him when he is not eating, so there is a clear difference in your attention and interaction when he *is* eating.

7. If your child should tantrum or become upset during a meal, first tell him "No!" firmly. Then if he continues, ignore him by turning away from him (or turning his chair away from the table) and do not talk to or about him during Time Out. This should last about 30-60 seconds. However, do not let his tantrums allow him to escape from doing something he is required to do (in other words, if tantrums are a way to escape eating, then placing him in Time Out will encourage tantrums since Time Out is more desirable than eating).

8. If you have any questions or problems, call the office at 335-1104.

Linda K. Hurley, Ph.D.
Licensed Psychologist
Pediatric and Child Clinical Psychology

deep breathing," "record each time Johnny sat on the toilet for 5 minutes") and helps the clinician review the child's (and parents') progress at future sessions. It also informs the participants that therapy is not something to be done for 1 hour per week in someone's office, but rather something to be practiced daily and reported on during the therapy hour.

Cognitive behavioral assignments are useful with older children and adolescents in individual therapy ("write down situations that triggered your angry feelings, what thoughts you had, and how you responded") and can be used to help the child make changes during subsequent therapy sessions (Wilkes et al., 1994). Before sending a child away with homework, the clinician should discuss what is expected, make sure the child understands what he or she is to do, and state any contingencies ("remember, we will play a game at the end of the session on the days you bring back your completed homework"). If contingencies were stated, they must be followed. The clinician should write down what he or she and the child agreed on in the chart and, if needed, write a contract for both the clinician and the child to sign.

Targeted Symptom Treatments

There is excellent research on the effectiveness of targeted behavioral interventions for specific childhood problems, including encopresis, enuresis, negative behaviors, school problems, and sleep problems. Carolyn Schroeder and Betty Gordon (1991), for example, have documented the effectiveness of some of these short-term protocols in a primary care setting, and a number of other resources have documented treatment effectiveness in a variety of settings (Matson, 1988; Ollendick, King, & Yule, 1994; Reynolds & Johnston, 1994; Roberts, 1995; Walker & Roberts, 1992).

OFFICE OVERHEAD

For practitioners working in a private practice setting, the issue of office costs will become more and more important as they accept more managed care referrals. Since reimbursement rates are lower and incomes tend to drop with increases in managed care patients, it will be necessary to reduce office expenses to the lowest practical level. This may mean negotiating for lower office rent, joining with others in a group to purchase supplies or services, or even forming groups with other psychologists or mental health professionals to share office expenses (e.g., for secretarial support, phone answering). An increase in managed care in an area will likely give rise to more group practices and fewer solo independent practices.

Based on estimates for other professionals, office overhead for psychologists should be approximately 38–40%. This means that psychologists should net about 60% after overhead expenses are paid (rent, insurance, secretarial help, supplies, utilities, and all similar expenses). This figure is based on estimates for physicians, since figures for psychologists were not available. It should be noted that as income increases, overhead percentage should decrease. Forty percent should be considered the maximum overhead amount for a successful practice.

HELPING CONSUMERS MAKE INFORMED CHOICES

Following publication of the widely discussed issue on effectiveness of therapy, *Consumer Reports* published an extensive review of managed care plans, with at least a nod to mental health coverage in these plans (Consumers Union, 1996). It is not unusual, in our experience, for patients or potential patients to call a psychologist when their employer's "open season" allows them to change health insurance plans and seek advice on which plan to choose. Of course, that decision is as individual as which clothes to wear to the office, and what is a good choice for one consumer may not be the right choice for another. Still, the clinician is in a powerful position to influence consumer behavior at that time.

As noted throughout this book, at times the publicity literature from an HMO may appear to promise to the consumer more than actually is available. Managed care plans often tout their HEDIS or NCQA ratings as "proof" that they are a good plan, but these measures are insufficient to measure quality and are sometimes misleading. For example, the NCQA accreditation does not look at outcome or satisfaction, but rather systems and processes. These are important factors to examine, but not the only ones. Consumers who are ill and use their health care coverage more often tend to rate managed care plans much differently than healthy consumers. Access to care becomes a more critical issue when the care is really needed. When mental health benefits are available, but not needed, they are always adequate. However, when a child needs an extensive assessment battery or therapy for a severe trauma, the limits of coverage suddenly become quite clear.

Rather than simply relaying one's experience with a managed care plan, it may be more effective for the clinician to help parents read the mental health benefits of the plans they are considering and see how they would fit into actual use. For example, if a plan covers 50% of up to $50 per session, the clinician can translate that figure into real dollars that the parent will have to pay out of pocket. Even though a parent may end up paying more out-of-pocket for one plan than another, if they have more choice over providers and services, it may be well worth it. One must keep in mind that managed care prefers medication over therapy, generally, and for some parents, this is not acceptable. The APA and other professional organizations have been increasing their efforts to educate consumers (for their own plans and for their employers) about what to request in managed care plans. Perhaps the easiest way to access this information is through the World Wide Web (http://www.apa.org; http://epn.org/families.html; http://www.medscape.com).

ADVOCATING FOR AND WITH CONSUMERS

Children and families require universal access to comprehensive, coordinated, and high-quality mental health services designed to address their unique needs. These services should combine prevention, early intervention, and treatment modalities and should be available across a range of community settings where children and families are traditionally served (APA Practice Directorate, 1996). Originally, HMOs were viewed as a way in which comprehensive health care (physical and mental) could be provided to greater numbers of people. The rise in health care costs minimized this view, such that HMOs and other managed care arrangements often have cost containment as the primary goal instead of improving service accessibility. Some commentators claim that managed care overall does extend service to those who may be unlikely to receive assistance in any other way. The clinician who takes the "higher road" of advocating for the best welfare of child patients and families serves several professional purposes. That is, clinicians are in a *profession*; one aspect of being a professional is rising above personal interests to advocate for those in need. The clinician cannot accomplish this, however, if he or she cannot maintain himself or herself in business. We believe that advocacy for children and families has several pay-offs, including the more self-serving ones of providing income for the clinician. In this section we describe settings where clinician's advocacy can improve children's services *and*, not coincidentally, create niches for clinical service delivery.

Within the School System

Outpatient mental health care can be provided within school settings by appropriately trained personnel. Schools already provide some services and may have on-staff school psychologists to provide some psychometric and academic assistance. Some school districts have mental health professionals available for therapeutic interventions, but this is not the norm. Greater demands are being placed on school systems to provide mental health services in addition to those required for academic placement. As the demand outstrips the capacity of school psychologists to provide therapy *and* educational services to children with DSM-IV diagnoses, for example, child specialty clinicians will be called on to consult and provide such services. Within these entry points, services can and should be provided, including direct and indirect services, consultation, and in-service training. Psychologists and other mental health clinicians can meet many of the needs of children and families in a coordinated, responsive manner when such services are managed and coordinated appropriately. The burden on schools to assess children's educational and developmental needs is increasing as managed care is limiting or denying coverage for these issues. By law, schools are required to provide appropriate assessment and intervention for these childhood concerns under many circumstances. One of us (LKH) has found that schools frequently tell parents that they cannot or will not do these assessments, and the managed care company also refuses to cover such testing, leaving parents frustrated and confused. The clinician can help parents obtain materials clearly defining their rights and help them advocate with the school district and/or managed care organization to provide what is needed for their child when that service is, in fact, covered by one entity or the other. Many school districts publish plain language guides to parents' and children's legal rights, and there are a number of advocacy agencies that help parents obtain covered services when their school district refuses. Unfortunately, no such advocacy organizations exist, to our knowledge, for obtaining coverage from managed care. However, legal remedies are still available when justified.

The other author (MCR) recently was approached by a school district to help set up a therapeutic classroom for children who were diagnosed as having serious emotional disorders and who needed an educational setting for assessment and therapy as they transitioned into regular classrooms. The therapeutic requirements could not be handled by an already overextended school psychology staff. These types of interactions with schools may create new niches for the child clinician outside of the managed care environment.

Primary Health Care Settings

More and more psychologists are establishing clinical practices within or affiliated with pediatric or other primary health care groups. These can assist in gaining referrals (within or outside of a managed care plan). Several models exist for these kinds of pediatric psychology practices (e.g., Hurley, 1995; Schroeder 1996; Schroeder & Gordon, 1991). The applications of pediatric psychology have been well documented (e.g., Roberts, 1995) for many medical conditions (e.g., encopresis) and the psychological concomitants of medical conditions (e.g., regimen adherence, psychosocial adjustment to chronic illness). If the clinician has the expertise, expanding this niche may fill a practice, even outside managed care.

At one time in his career, one of us (MCR) developed a reputation for treating encopresis based on a series of embarrassed whispered referrals among parents for "kids that had trouble pooping." As a result many patients were seen (and not one filed an insurance claim). Psychosocial programs for children and families with special health care needs (e.g., children with cancer) can be developed by the clinician by seeking funding from charitable organizations (e.g., Junior League, churches) or a self-pay system from parents. For example, Schroeder and Gordon (1991) described some of their pediatric practice's groups and workshops.

Prevention

Prevention services for mental health should be as accessible as basic physical health prevention services, such as immunizations. These prevention services could be included in health care reform initiatives. If such services are provided for physical health, then they should be provided for mental health. There is some debate as to whether any such services should be paid for out of public funds, but when they are, mental health should be on par with physical health services.

Chapter 7 includes an extensive discussion of medical cost offset and the justification for treating mental disorders as a cost savings mechanism.

Flexible Funding for Alternative Services

Alternative services, including home-based clinical and prevention services, group therapy, and "wrap-around" programs provide comprehensive, individually tailored services and family preservation initiatives. These approaches utilize cross-disciplinary and cross-setting funding (Behar et al., 1996). The concepts of a continuum of care include a fully integrated range of serve availability, including crisis interventions, clinical case management, outpatient and day treatment, and more intensive services such as group homes and hospitalization. As states have increasingly privatized Medicaid, agencies and groups of clinicians have obtained contracts for various service components. As the mental health and public welfare field has moved in this direction, careful research and policy advocacy are needed to consider the impact (Bickman et al., 1995). In some instances, funding may be flexibly available to cover what needs to be done. Indeed, the original concept of continuum of care encompassed flexible funding. However, as it has been implemented in many states, regulations are rigidly applied to restrict innovation and fully integrated coverage.

Integrated Mental Health Services for Children

Coordination and interagency collaboration for care of children and families must be structured and appropriately funded for maximum effectiveness. Emphasis on these systems of care will allow for more integrated services, which are accessible, comprehensive, consumer-driven, outcome-oriented, and focused on competence strengthening. At the present time, managed care does not generally cover such services for children, although state systems are presumably moving in this direction with privatization of Medicaid services. Clinicians can advocate for changes in policy and law in order to mandate that such services for children be covered by their health insurance.

CHANGING THE MENTAL HEALTH CARE SYSTEM

In 1996, approximately 8 million American children suffered from a mental disorder. Even more would have benefited from mental health interventions for medical or developmental problems. To encourage cost-effective treatment, a broad array of services, including inpatient, outpatient, and residential services, must be available and accessible to those who need it. Research clearly shows that outpatient treatment is more cost-effective than inpatient treatment, so benefit plans should be designed to encourage less costly alternatives to inpatient treatment, where appropriate, without putting patients or others at risk. This benefit design should be based on the following tenets:

- The least restrictive appropriate care setting should be the treatment of choice, with inpatient services provided only to those with the most serious disorders. When patients need inpatient care, the amount of care should be based on actual need rather than arbitrary limits.
- People with serious mental illness need mental health treatment that includes long-term care sufficient to meet their needs.
- Patients should have the flexibility to trade inpatient and outpatient benefits as well as coverage for nonhospital-based services such as day treatment, school-based programs, residential treatment, and partial hospitalization.
- The patient's or family's ability to pay should be considered in setting copayments. Where needed, copayments should be subsidized to avoid limiting access or financial hardship when individuals need treatment. Research has shown that both inpatient and outpatient utilization of mental health services can be controlled by copayments, deductibles, and proper benefit design, and this has been further demonstrated by real-life experiences of businesses and corporations.
- The confidentiality and welfare of consumers should be protected by provisions and safeguards included in benefit plans and/or state laws.
- Funding initiatives should support the training of psychologists and other mental health professionals so there is sufficient care for the poor and underserved, especially in rural and inner-city areas.
- Psychologists should work toward collaborative relationships with primary care providers.
- The public mental health system should be designed and used to provide services to individuals and communities who might not otherwise have access to such services.
- Behavioral research on health promotion, disease prevention, and treatment efficacy should be adequately funded because that is the basis of a cost-efficient health care system (APA Practice Directorate, 1996).

Psychologists interested in advocacy within their state and at the national level can use these suggestions to promote a better health care delivery system by working with their state and local psychological associations, and advocating with business and consumer groups for these changes. The APA has a great deal of supportive literature available, which is updated frequently to address those issues currently before Congress and the state legislatures.

ADAPTING TO MANAGED CARE

We view the phrase "adapting to managed care" as an accurate way to view the *process* of change, while maintaining professional standards and making a decent living. Adapting is not an all-or-none, once-and-for-all time phenomenon—it is ongoing in finding ways to do what needs to be done within certain parameters. A clinician need not "cave in" to all aspects of managed care in order to survive in this adaptation process. Over time, we expect managed care as a movement will also adapt—to consumers' demands for accessibility and quality services and to professional concerns over ethical and competent practice. How this reciprocal adaptation takes place is not likely to be productive with antagonistic and shrill confrontation, but from a careful effort to document needs for and benefits of mental health services provided by qualified clinicians. One commentator has predicted that, by the year 2000, 50% of private practice psychologists will be out of business (Cummings, 1995, 1996). This prediction need not come true for those clinicians willing to adapt to managed care, while not abandoning principled practice. Yet, it is certain that a complete return to earlier systems of insurance reimbursement and care coordination will not occur.

Limiting Negative Impact of Managed Care on a Clinical Child/Pediatric Psychology Practice

A child/pediatric psychologist opened a private practice in a medium-sized metropolitan area. She was one of a very few psychologists with specialty training in child clinical/pediatric psychology and was able to get on several managed care panels. One particular company, Managed Care Plan H (MCPH), the largest managed care company in the area, provided her with more referrals than she could handle. After several months, the psychologist's waiting list became so long that physicians and other referral sources quit referring to her. She began getting most of her business directly through referrals from MCPH. After one year, MCPH decided to cut their reimbursement rates by 20%. This was quite a blow to the psychologist's income, but was tolerable, since the volume of business was so high. The MCPH business she saw rose to over 50% of her practice. One day, she received a notice that MCPH was dropping their reimbursement for psychologists to just 50% of her usual charges within 30 days. Calculating her overhead costs, the psychologist realized that she would be losing money if she continued in this system at these new rates. Therefore, she considered resigning from MCPH, but she would likely take a 50% cut in income if she dropped off the MCPH panel. However, if she stayed on MCPH, she would still see almost a 40% drop in income from those patients. In addition, her regular referral sources had dried up because of her overinvolvement with MCPH.

The solution to the above dilemma is not an easy one. In fact, the psychologist did drop MCPH and her income did drop tremendously. She had to do extensive marketing, find other sources of income, and try to fix a very badly broken practice. The purpose of this chapter is to help clinicians avoid getting in such a situation.

ADVANTAGES AND DISADVANTAGES OF PRACTICING IN A MANAGED CARE ENVIRONMENT

Most of us would agree that change is difficult. Therefore, adapting to managed care requirements is probably more challenging to established clinicians who have already become comfortable with their own particular style of business and clinical practice. For some, the fact of their long-established practice, reliable referrals, and nearness to retirement will lead them to opt out of managed care practice. For those just starting out, entering the managed care market may be easier because there will be no long-set patterns to change. However, those who have been in practice for 5–20 years probably face the greatest amount of change in terms of income, practice patterns, and business practices. In considering whether and how to enter the managed care marketplace, one must keep in mind that this is a business decision, and the relationship between the clinician and the managed care entity is a business relationship. As noted in Chapter 3, clinicians need to pay careful attention to the business and legal aspects of each managed care relationship and carefully consider the advantages and disadvantages of each *before* signing on as a provider.

Advantages

A primary advantage in becoming a managed care provider is the likelihood of increased referrals and a larger patient base. Indeed, as managed care arrangements penetrate deeper and wider into public and private services, the sources of patients for practitioners will become more and more restricted. In some areas of the country, managed care, in some form or another, has locked in a sizeable majority of the insured population. This control may limit the clinician's autonomy and income to some degree, but it may also serve to funnel a larger proportion of referrals not available to the clinician previously through other marketing strategies. The managed care organization will often provide some free advertising and marketing by publishing the provider's name and other information in their directory. Being on a provider panel, however, does not guarantee that any one clinician will receive a particular number of referrals. In fact, some managed care organizations sign on so many providers initially in a locality that it is largely up to the provider to market his or her availability within that system to referral sources.

Another possible advantage of being on a managed care panel is that billing may be simplified and payment may be facilitated. Billing is simplified only if the clinician also bills other insurance plans. Simplified billing may be no more than a managed care company public relationships pretense, unfortunately, because many clinicians experience considerable difficulty in completing the paperwork to file a claim, tracking it through the system, and actually getting full payment in a timely manner. Many companies have provider relations representatives whose purpose is to ease these problems, but they, too, take time and effort to access. In some managed care systems, the payment process is truly facilitated, but at professional meetings and in publications, the payment problem remains a significant sore point for clinicians (see Cantor, 1997). In outpatient practices, clinicians often expect or require full payment at the time service is rendered, even though they may assist patients in filing their own insurance claims. In this case, billing becomes more complicated, and the clinician must adjust to waiting for payments while claims are processed, refiled, and reprocessed.

Being on one managed care panel may facilitate joining other panels. Becoming a full-time employee of an HMO may provide benefits such as predictable income or salary and insurance benefits that must be purchased independently in a private practice. In addition, one may also benefit from affiliation with other health care professionals (Higuchi, 1994).

Disadvantages

As previously mentioned, billing may become easier or more complicated, depending on the previous practice. Billing for services adds cost to the provision of services, and the cost of billing is often not factored into the clinician's business cost estimate. Most managed care contracts provide for payment within a certain number of days, or payment will revert to the provider's full fee. However, in practice, this additional fee may be difficult and expensive to collect. If the clinician employs a billing service that charges by the hour, the billing service charge may equal or exceed the additional amount collected from the managed care entity. One of us (LKH) has had the experience of one managed care plan being 2 years behind in payment of claims. This relationship ended up requiring legal action to collect the amounts due. Obviously, hiring an attorney to assist in collections is quite costly and can only be justified when amounts owed are quite large. Postponement of payments is a frequent complaint. Sometimes these are imposed through inefficient procedures, deliberate delays, or financial turmoil within a plan.

Another disadvantage of working with a managed care organization is the usual requirement to agree to accept a discounted payment from what the clinician usually charges (ranging from a 25–50% discount or more). Most typically, payments to providers continue to be reduced even more as managed care plans evolve generation by generation. This can be quite devastating to a clinical practice as illustrated in this chapter's opening vignette.

Additionally, withholding a portion of the payment can create a significant cash flow problem (with a portion of each fee withheld until the end of a business year when the plan balances its books). In an open letter to a managed care company published in the *APA Monitor*, Dorothy Cantor (1997) strongly protested the further reduction of the already discounted fee in the contract without advance notification or permission. She articulated that "I am confident that as more people become aware of the outrageous behavior of managed mental health-care companies, public pressure will force changes in the way in which these services are being rationed" (p. 2).

Most HMO and PPO plans will allow only a limited number of sessions per year, but that number is frequently reduced even further by the utilization review process. This reduction in service to a patient in psychological need can potentially cause ethical and legal problems (see Chapter 3 and Higuchi, 1994). The costs of additional documentation, (often required in managed care plans) and potentially unreimbursed service (sometimes required ethically for the patient's care) are absorbed by the provider. These become other, largely unexpected, business expenses. These types of expenses are generally not tax-deductible and must simply be absorbed. This issue highlights again the need for the clinician to determine, in advance of signing a contract, whether the managed care plan requires preauthorization for services and whether the clinician is allowed to bill the patient for any disallowed services (which may be restricted or denied by the managed care contract).

DIVERSIFY—BALANCING SOURCES OF MANAGED CARE REIMBURSEMENT

Monitoring Managed Care Income

A clinician may become tempted to become "*the*" provider for a large, well-paying managed care company, and in many cases, clinicians who specialize in child psychology can have a lucrative "niche market." Various writers have recommended limiting managed care reimbursement to 40–50% of a practice income ("Managed Care," 1994), but we also suggest a prudent business practice is to limit exposure in any *single* managed care entity to less than or equal to 15% of income. That is the maximum amount of income most psychologists can afford to risk in a precipitous income loss, should the managed care company drop them as a provider, go bankrupt, be merged or bought out, or reduce reimbursement to untenable rates. In addition, we recommend that a clinician in a solo practice or small group limit total managed care sources to 60% or less of overall practice income for the same reasons. Others suggest keeping managed care income to 30–40% of total practice income. Some large group practices are structured in such a way that they can accommodate a greater percentage of managed care income and can tolerate greater risk, but most independent or small group practices cannot. In order to achieve this balance, clinicians must find other sources of income outside of managed care. The clinician may wish to consult his or her accountant and local area professional organization on this issue.

To diversify sources of managed care income, obviously the clinician must join multiple managed care panels. However, caution must be exercised in doing this. As stated in Chapter 3, the clinician would not be wise to join any panels without carefully reading contracts and researching the companies with which he or she is considering developing a business relationship and consulting an attorney if needed. Nonetheless, the presumed benefits of joining several *good* managed care panels include the ability to decrease one's dependence on any single source of income.

Of course, in order to track sources of income, clinicians must carefully document their activities. Boxes 5.1a and 5.1b are examples of a form for tracking managed care income and a blank form to use. Many computerized billing programs can automatically print out such information as income by payer, number of patients by payer, and similar business practice data. This type of program is likely to be a time-saver as well as a valuable business tool for those who have access to such equipment. We recommend that the clinician carefully consider the information provided by such software programs before purchasing one.

It is difficult to diversify sources of managed care income unless the clinician can get on provider panels. Clinicians are often informed that a managed care company's panel is "full" and that they will not accept any new applications. One clinician reported being informed that it would be at least 3 years before the plan anticipated opening their panel to new applicants!

Diversifying Income Sources

In addition to diversifying within the managed care system, the clinician can also diversify the income sources for the overall practice. Adding contracts, such as from school districts, group homes, outpatient medical clinics, or community agencies, can add dependable income. Most contracts are for a set fee in

BOX 5.1a. SAMPLE TRACKING FORM FOR MANAGED CARE ACCOUNTS

Managed Care Company A

Patient name	Dates of visits	Diagnoses	# Approved visits	Service code	Payment rate	Date billed	Date paid	Correct amount?	Action
Andrews, John	1/10/96	r/o 300.40	1	90801	$130	1/13/96	2/10/96	y	
	1/17/96	300.40	5	90844	$78	1/23/96	2/20/96	y	
	1/23/96	300.40		90844	$78	1/23/96	2/20/96	n	resubmit
Smith, Susan	1/6/96	r/o314.01, r/o313.81	3	90801	$130	1/7/96	2/5/96	y	
	1/10/96	r/o314.01, r/o313.81	6 hrs	90830	$98/hr	1/13/96	2/10/96	n	paid for 1hr only; resubmit
	1/17/96	314.01; 313.81		90844	$78	1/23/96	2/20/96	y	
	1/23/96	314.01; 313.81		90844	$78	1/23/96	2/20/96	n	resubmit

BOX 5.1b. BLANK TRACKING FORM FOR MANAGED CARE ACCOUNTS

Managed Care Company A: _____   Phone Number: _____

Provider Relations Contact Person: _____

Patient name	Dates of visits	Diagnoses	# Approved visits	Service code	Payment rate	Date billed	Date paid	Correct amount?	Action

exchange for a certain number of hours per week or month (and may require some availability for nonreimbursed consultation). The clinician must balance the cost and effort of providing these services with this additional and reliable income to make it worthwhile. For example, it may not be cost-effective to drive 30 minutes each way to do a 2-hour per week contract. If it can be arranged, the contract or consultantship may be more worthwhile to do 2 half-days per month, or even a full day per month at the same rate. The clinician must calculate travel time and expenses in accepting a contract (which will be for less than the usual hourly rate but it would be reliable income). The income can form the base of finances necessary to maintain a practice as well as withstand the vicissitudes of managed care. If the contracted work can be scheduled in normally open hours not taken by patients (e.g., first thing in the morning), then there is no loss of prime session time for child patients (e.g., after school hours).

Teaching Groups

Clinicians can also participate in teaching groups for a reduced fee, which will provide some income but will also likely be a source of additional referrals to the clinical practice. Groups offered on such topics as "Managing the Strong-Willed Child," "Tips for Helping Children Adjust to Stepfamilies," and "Sex Education for School-Aged Children—How to Tell, What to Tell" can be big practice enhancers. In Chapter 6, we discuss practice enhancers such as parent education groups and classes that can be used by a clinician to market clinical services and develop referral sources outside managed care panels.

EVALUATING THE BUSINESS, PROTECTING THE PRACTICE: LETHAL PITFALLS TO AVOID

As previously stated, clinicians must ensure that their practices are not overbalanced by a single managed care entity. The only way to do this is to regularly evaluate practice income. Computerized billing programs or billing services may be able to print out the percentage of business generated from each managed care company with which the clinician contracts and can also report the overall amount of income from managed care versus other sources (private pay, contracts, etc.). In Chapter 6, Boxes 6.1 and 6.2 provide forms for the clinician to use in tracking sources of income and practice patterns. Clinicians should check these figures at least quarterly to make changes in the payer mix as needed. The goal of having less than 60% of one's income from all managed care sources (and no more than 15% from any one such source) is much easier said than done. However, for the solo practitioner or small group, we suggest it may be critical to survival.

HANDLING INSURANCE CLAIMS

The process of filing health insurance claims and the insurance company's payment procedures can have a significant impact on the financial health of a clinician's practice. Reviewing how claims are handled and processed in the clinician's office can help determine whether changes are needed. The two basic systems for filing claims are manual and electronic, or computer-filed, claims.

In offices (or particular cases) where claims are filed manually, each patient should complete an information form at the initial visit that includes all the information needed by the clinician to submit the claims. This form should be updated periodically (at least once per year) for longer-term patients, as information such as address or insurance coverage may change. The patient should be asked about current insurance coverage at least once per month, and copies of insurance/Medicare/Medicaid eligibility statements should be updated in the claims file as needed. Electronic claims filing is often the desired method of filing claims; insurance companies often prefer this method and will generally promise quicker reimbursement for such claims. Providers must be sure they understand the computer specifications and requirements associated with automated claims submission. The effort of learning various intricate systems pays off only if used repeatedly. Additionally, confirmation of receipt of a claim will help the clinician track its processing. Some companies rely on faxed claims (and other patient history data). Both electronic or faxed submission requires careful overview to protect patient confidentiality. (This caveat applies to regular mail, but the ramifications seem greater with the newer forms of information transfer.)

Collection policies vary from carrier to carrier, but most require that a managed care provider collect the required copayment from the patient or insured parent. Although some carriers acknowledge that there may be circumstances affecting a patient's ability to pay, Medicare, for example, generally considers it fraud for a provider not to collect these copayments. While it may be a common practice for some offices to "write off" the copayment, the clinician is responsible for understanding the insurance company's rules regarding this in order to avoid problems later.

Claims forms must be completed fully, accurately, and legibly for claims to be paid in a timely fashion. The forms required often vary from carrier to carrier, and it is essential to use the correct form. Although this would seem to require no emphasis, we know of several clinicians who could not collect on claims because of the wrong form or incomplete information. The clinician must be certain that the appropriate procedure and diagnosis codes are used for all services and that information regarding each visit is substantiated in the patient record. A regular schedule for submitting claims will help a business run more smoothly. Claims should be filed weekly or at the very least, every other week.

The clinician can establish a "suspense file" or other reminder method to inquire regularly about the status of unpaid claims. These inquiries should usually be done within 1 month after filing. When unpaid claims are not investigated or pursued by the clinician, they often remain unpaid. If an insurance company rejects a claim, the clinician should not simply accept the carrier's decision. He or she should review the claim to determine whether there have been any errors in coding or other inaccuracies or omissions. After correcting any errors, a standard letter asking for reconsideration of the claim should be sent, or a phone call placed to the claims department. Any phone calls ought to be documented with the insurance representative's name, date and time of the call, and a summary of the call. The clinician should ask for any promises to pay to be sent in writing. Then the clinician should follow up with a letter verifying the conversation. If a claim is denied a second time, the clinician may need to consider invoking his or her right to appeal as set out in the contract or provider relations information. It is not uncommon, in our experience, for claims to be repeatedly refiled, rejected, and further investigated before they are finally paid.

Insurance claims are all too frequently underpaid. To avoid this income loss, the clinician needs to regularly review submissions and payments for any discrepancies. Since reimbursement rates vary not only from carrier to carrier, but even within carriers from plan to plan, this can be a daunting task. A master file of reimbursement rates for various contracts can be maintained in order to make these reviews more efficient (see Box 5.2 for an example). The clinician must determine which underpaid claims are worth resubmitting. Frequently occurring but small underpayments or very large claims with significant underpayment are often worth the effort. When a billing service has been engaged, the clinician should check the service's policy on refiling incorrectly paid claims. Many services will automatically resubmit all claims that are incorrectly paid, no matter how small the amount, especially when the billing service is being paid on a percentage of collections basis. The cost of such effort versus the return must be calculated. Frequent (and seemingly deliberate) underpayments are signs of poor business practices on the part of the managed care companies. Depending on the clinician's ability to withstand being unceremoniously dropped from a panel, vigorous protest may be called for to the company itself (as illustrated by Cantor, 1997), to the Better Business Bureau, and to the state insurance commissioner. (As we note elsewhere, being dropped from a panel for asserting rights set out in the provider contract is both objectionable and actionable legally.)

Clinicians should make a habit of reviewing newsletters and publications from insurance carriers for changes in codes and reimbursement policies that apply to mental health services. Any changes that affect the clinician's practice should be noted in the billing file or sent to the billing service used by the practice.

BOX 5.2. EXAMPLE OF RECORDING FORM FOR REIMBURSEMENT RATES BY MANAGED CARE PLANS

Managed Care Company	Plan name	Procedure code	Copayment	Total rate of reimbursement
TangoPlus	PrimoUltra	90801	$30	$130
		90830	n/a	n/a
		90844	$20	$68
	BonFrere	90801	$10	$100
	Dynamo	90830	$10	$ 90/hr
		90844	$10	$ 70
Alpha Systems	Bond-Med	90801	20%	$120
Supreme		90830	20%	$110/hr
		90844	20% first five visits	$ 98
			50% sixth–twelfth visit	$ 98

MARKETING

Marketing within a Managed Care Company

Managed care organizations provide some minimal marketing for the providers on their panels by listing provider names in the plan's directory. However, it is generally necessary for clinicians to do additional marketing themselves to obtain patients covered under a plan, unless they are employed in a full-time position within a managed care organization. There are several approaches to marketing, all of which can be beneficial to the practice in general. As we discuss throughout this book, marketing may take different forms. Some differences may be required depending on the clinician's locale and circumstances.

Marketing to Primary Care

Primary care physicians can be an excellent source of referrals, whether or not one's practice is within a primary care setting. One commentator stated that physicians, nearly as much as the public, need to be educated regarding the distinction between the various mental health providers and how psychologists can be integrated into their practice models (Carr, 1996). He further suggests that the clinician should illustrate how his or her unique services are applicable in a primary care setting. For the child psychologist, this demonstration may include such things as the effective treatment of encopresis or bed-wetting, assessment of attention problems, and similar complaints that fill a pediatrician's day but that he or she does not have the time or interest to fully deal with.

The second part of the education process in primary care, according to Carr (1996), is to help physicians understand how to access one's skills. We would add that it is also important to educate nurses and office staff. This process will likely involve repetition of the information on a number of occasions. The probability of receiving referrals is increased when the physician, nurses, and staff know not only one's name, but also what the clinician does and how to get a patient to the clinician for services.

Maintaining Contact with Referral Sources

Reaching these goals requires a commitment to maintaining contact with one's referral sources (and potential referral sources). Carr (1996) suggests several useful strategies:

1 | Prepare handouts that explain the clinician's approach to common problems, highlighting any special techniques or skills one has. These same handouts may be helpful in dealing with the media or with insurance companies as one tries to explain why treatment is needed and what the reasonable expectations for outcome are. (Examples of these are depicted in Boxes 6.1 and 6.2; we discuss various topics and formats for these handouts in Chapter 6).

2 | The clinician can prepare a guide for the primary care office listing the steps involved in referring to the clinician. This guide can include suggestions on how to explain to the patient the referral to a psychologist and even a sample letter, explaining how a psychologist can help with their child's problem, which can be copied and given to patients. Providing a potential patient with an overview of the clinician and his or her practice can help ensure that the patient makes and keeps an appointment.

3 | In all cases, but particularly when working with physicians, the clinician should emphasize his or her availability and accessibility. One of the main complaints primary care physicians have with many members of the psychiatry profession is that it takes too long: too

long to get a consultation, to get a call returned, to see progress, to get feedback. When a referral is made, the clinician should see the patient in a timely manner and should communicate with the referring physician as soon as possible. With the patient's permission, an initial letter acknowledging the referral and summarizing the proposed treatment plan should be sent as soon as the patient has been seen. If treatment continues over an extended period, occasional updates should also be sent, if the referring physician requests it and the patient agrees. When treatment is terminated, a treatment summary letter should be sent, with a note of thanks for the referral.

Finally, we emphasize that an important way to maintain contact and communicate professionalism is through the use of a Referral Source Satisfaction Questionnaire (an example is presented in Box 4.7 in Chapter 4).

Public and Business Educational Campaigns

Sullivan (1996) reported on an effort by the Rhode Island Psychological Association (RIPA) to educate business leaders about the value of psychological services. They called their outreach effort "Campaign for Care." The effort was started when a psychologist became fed up with the massive amount of paperwork required to authorize minimal amounts of treatment. Dr. Patricia Raymond, the psychologist who spearheaded the campaign, developed a multidisciplinary mental health coalition to approach employers and business leaders directly at a Chamber of Commerce event. In addition, RIPA developed their own high-quality brochure called *Peace of Mind: Buying Mental Health Insurance for Your Company* to assist employers in purchasing mental health insurance for their companies. The brochure clearly explains benefit design and cost-containment practices. An accompanying card delineated the principles of good mental health insurance coverage, including such items as, "Allow a minimum of 10 unmanaged outpatient psychotherapy visits each calendar year," and "Have a schedule of copayments that increases in steps so that your employees share an increasing portion of the cost the longer they are in treatment."

This effort is similar and very much in concert with the APA's Public Education Campaign, "Talk to Someone Who Can Help." The positive results experienced by the Rhode Island group indicates the need for psychologists to talk directly to business leaders about mental health services and how appropriate insurance coverage can benefit their businesses. Although such a sizable campaign is not something that could be undertaken by a single individual, state or local psychological associations can be tapped for resources and support in such an effort. In addition, APA will provide information and support, through the Practice Directorate, to groups wishing to support the Public Education Campaign. (See Chapter 2 for information on contacting the Practice Directorate offices.)

POS OPTION

A point-of-service (POS) option allows a patient to choose any provider who is willing to accept the provisions of a particular managed care plan, generally including discounted fees, preauthorization, UR, and similar provisions. Many states have passed POS statutes requiring managed care plans to offer such alternatives. Congress is currently considering requiring all managed care companies to offer POS options and other patient safeguards. The availability of a POS option can avoid disruption in service caused when a patient's insurance benefits change or when a provider drops off or is dropped from a panel but the patient needs to continue seeing a particular clinician for a period of time.

GROUP PRACTICE

For clinicians who choose to make managed care a significant part of their practice, joining other providers in a group practice can decrease the risks and maximize the benefits of managed care. There are several types of groups or networks, many of which are formed for the primary purpose of contracting with managed care organizations. Group practices have the advantages of being more attractive to third-party payers, combining administrative functions, decreasing costs, and providing internal quality assurance and utilization management. It is more efficient for large payers and networks to contract with a single group capable of providing all the covered benefits offered than to contract with numerous small groups and individuals (Yenney & APA Practice Directorate, 1994). A group has the advantage of being able to offer more diverse services and longer hours. Managed care organizations prefer groups because they are more able than solo providers to accept discounted fees or capitated payments to treat very large patient pools (Schachner, 1994).

Advantages

In addition to the benefits mentioned in the last section, there are several specific advantages for managed care companies, patients, and providers to being in a group practice:

■ Administrative costs are reduced because the managed care company has fewer billing and tax ID numbers to contend with and referrals are made to one group that can provide a broad range of services. Groups generally provide their own internal peer review and quality assurance.

■ Multispecialty groups offer the advantage of getting the patient to the right provider quickly, even if the initial referral to one provider is not appropriate.

■ Groups tend to be better able to adapt to the efficiencies of electronic processing demands of managed care organizations.

■ Group practices may become large enough and efficient enough to contract directly with employers and health insurance purchasers, thus cutting out the cost of the managed care middleman (Schachner, 1994).

Disadvantages

As in all of life, group practice also has its down side for the various parties, including:

■ Necessity of compromise on a number of issues ranging from which bank to use to how much to charge in fees. Individuals may need to change pension plans, malpractice carriers, accountants, and other aspects of business practice. The professional relationships developed while in independent practice may have to be put aside in favor of ones the group chooses. The group's choice of pension plans may be significantly better or worse than the individual's plan and may lead to significant tax ramifications.

■ Thinking *as a group* can be difficult for independent-minded clinicians. All members of the group will need to agree on the group's goals and mission. Otherwise, one person may undermine the efforts of the rest.

■ Limits on authority may be difficult for individuals to accept. The governing board of the group will make most decisions for the typical group. Clinicians should carefully examine how much power a board has before signing on and should feel comfortable allowing another entity, and the individuals who make up that entity, to make those decisions.

■ Hidden costs may decrease any savings that group membership may seem to imply. Some group practices may have hidden expenses, such as those from duplication of services. In addition, there may be additional administrative costs not present in a solo practice, such as office manager's or administrator's salaries and benefits. Of course, all of these expenses are paid for by the fees generated by the clinicians.

■ Greater exposure to liability: As a solo practitioner, the clinician has only himself or herself to worry about. But once a clinician joins a group, he or she has exposure to all the malpractice histories and potential actions of all the group members. If the corporation is sued, everyone's liability insurance rates may increase. Clinicians also face risk for uninsured liabilities over which they have no control, such as sexual harassment. As a small business, there can be problems finding health insurance for the whole group if one employee has a significant preexisting health condition. In addition, the financial risk of having to cover some uninsured costs of such an employee may be necessary for the small business to pay for in order to obtain group coverage.

■ Legal issues: Although antitrust laws have recently been revised and clarified, it is still an area that must be carefully examined in forming groups. There may be other state laws, such as self-referral prohibitions, that come into play in a group arrangement. Clinicians must seek expert legal advice to avoid liability risk as much as possible (Mangan, 1993).

TYPES OF GROUPS

The number and variety of group practices has grown as providers struggle to find ways to integrate managed care into their practices and to accommodate the changes in managed care systems as these entities evolved. Joining other clinicians to accept capitated contracts and deal with other managed care issues is one way to spread the financial risks more broadly. In addition, managed care organizations are looking for groups that can provide most or all services covered by their plans. Here, we will focus on those types of groups that were developed primarily for the purpose of contracting with managed care. In forming managed care groups, clinicians should be aware that their general professional liability insurance may not defend or protect them against claims of restraint of trade, price-fixing, or antitrust law violations.

The current focus in managed care is on integrated delivery systems, which basically provide "one-stop shopping" to consumers of mental health services. Purchasers of health insurance can contract with a single organization that provides a full continuum of care.

Independent Practice Association (IPA)

An IPA is an entity formed by independent practitioners for the purpose of contracting with managed care organizations. The IPA typically contracts with managed care plans to receive a capitated payment for those services offered through the IPA. The IPA contracts with individual clinicians to pay a discounted fee-for-service rate or a capitated rate (a specific amount per case, usually). IPAs are often formed by clinicians who have a business background and large amounts of capital, although they can at times be formed by clinicians with limited business experience in concert with business professionals who can provide the expertise needed to manage capitated contracts. An IPA is a legal entity organized and governed by individual clinicians for the purpose of collectively entering into contracts to provide services to enrolled populations. The contracts could include fee-for-service, discounted fee-for-service, capitation, or other options, depending on what the IPA negotiates with the plan purchaser.

State laws vary on who can form an IPA: In some states only same-profession partnerships are allowed, although they can generally hire other professionals. IPAs take time and money to develop. A significant amount of capital is typically invested by the principles in the group for the purpose of guaranteeing that services will be provided at the start and to allow for growth later on. For solo practitioners or those without access to the amount of capital required, joining an established IPA as a provider may be an option (Yenney & APA, 1994). IPAs are nonexclusive, so clinicians are free to contract with other groups and fee-for-service individuals. This "partial integration" allows providers to enter into managed care contracts while still retaining a degree of independence (Homchick, 1994).

Group Practice without Walls (GPWW or GWW)

A group practice without walls (GPWW) is a framework which allows individual clinicians (or small groups) to form a corporate relationship without moving in together. Each individual maintains his or her own individual office, and from the patient's perspective, there is little change. The clinicians most typically form a corporation or partnership that becomes their employer. This allows for a uniform fee schedule and a single tax ID and billing number. All revenues go into a common account that then pays the group's expenses and salaries. The clinician's salary is usually dependent on the individual's billings and collections.

GPWWs may save costs in one area, but often duplicate costs in another. For example, clinicians may save money by purchasing supplies in bulk, purchasing insurance as a group, and hiring a single billing service. However, there may be duplicated or underutilized services that can be costly, such as the need for a receptionist at every site. In a GPWW, the clinician typically has access to more sophisticated office management services than most individual clinicians have. Groups can negotiate contracts with volume purchasers, which may also benefit individual clinicians. Having geographically diverse offices has both pros and cons. On the one hand, the potential service area may be expanded, but on the other, it is more difficult to monitor the activities of the individual members. There are some state laws that affect a clinician's ability to refer to other clinicians within the group, and again it is necessary for potential GPWWs to seek legal advice before entering into a group arrangement.

Provider Hospital Organization (PHO)

A provider hospital organization (PHO) consists of at least one hospital and at least one provider group that form a network in order to contract with managed care plans. This model typically includes a wide variety of clinicians and specialties so that the group can truly offer the managed care plan a complete range of services, including inpatient and outpatient care, assessment, therapy, medication management, and other services. A PHO does not have to be a separate legal entity, and clinicians who join a PHO may continue to practice independently. Because laws vary from state to state regarding who can form such partnerships, it will be necessary to consult an attorney regarding these issues. PHOs have the advantage of access to greater capital through the hospital-partner, but clinicians will also be expected to contribute financially to the venture. Clinicians must be sure they understand and agree with the plans for how money will be spent. PHOs typically accept capitated contracts and then pay providers on either a fee-for-service or capitated basis. Withholds on fee payments are common, as in most cases where capitation contracts are accepted (Yenney & APA, 1994).

Antitrust Issues

Federal and most state antitrust laws can be a major legal issue for groups, particularly for IPAs. Recently, federal antitrust enforcement agencies issued revised policy guidelines that are more flexible as applied to provider networks. The new guidelines were published in August 1996 and address changes from the 1994 statements related to provider networks. The policy statements recognize that "by developing and implementing mechanisms that encourage physicians to collaborate in practicing efficiently," networks may "promise significant procompetitive benefits for consumers of health care services" ("New Anti-trust Guidelines," 1996). Presumably these collaborations include psychologists. The key to avoiding antitrust violations appears to lie in the concept of "safety zones" for joint pricing of services. "Safety zones" specify conditions under which provider networks can collaborate in establishing group policies (such as fee structures and billing practices) without violating federal anti-trust laws. These zones apply to provider networks that share substantial financial risk:

- Nonexclusive networks: Networks that account for less than or equal to 30% of the physicians with hospital staff privileges in a geographic market. Each specialty is considered separately.
- Exclusive networks: If providers are only allowed to contract with health plans through the network, the safety zone is 20% ("New Antitrust Guidelines," 1996).

To legally get around the antitrust issues while still maintaining the ability to set fees for contracts, some groups use the "messenger model." This model is most often used by networks that do not necessarily share substantial financial risk, but may still contract on a fee-for-service basis. Under the messenger model, a messenger goes back and forth between the various providers and a payer until a contract is agreed upon. The messenger cannot negotiate on behalf of the providers, cannot inform individual providers what the other providers have agreed or stated with respect to the proposed contract, cannot express an opinion regarding the contract, and cannot decide to withhold or convey the offer to providers. Individual clinicians are free to accept the contract and its provisions or decline to participate.

As can be seen from this brief discussion, legal issues can be quite tricky in group contracting. The clinician or group is advised to seek expert legal advice from an attorney who is well versed on these aspects of health care and mental health law.

CAPITATION

The current trend in managed mental health care is capitation. Capitation refers to contracts in which a provider group agrees to provide specific mental health services to a defined population of enrollees for a set monthly fee per patient (or sometimes a set fee per episode per patient). The provider group bears the risk that the cost of services may exceed the capitated payment. They manage this risk through stop-loss insurance, internal utilization review programs, and withholdings from providers' payments (Homchick, 1994). To accept and successfully manage capitation, psychologists must be able to predict their costs. Without this ability, the psychologist could not reasonably assume the risk that capitation entails (Cummings, 1995). The ability to absorb the risks posed by capitation may be difficult for an individual clinician.

Already, managed care organizations are offering psychiatrists capitated "per episode" payments of $300–$500 for psychiatric hospitalizations. Psychologists who plan to work in managed care need to educate themselves about capitation in order to pursue these contracts. As HMOs merge with managed mental health care plans, primary care physicians will have less reason to try to manage behavioral concerns in their offices and are likely to pass capitated patients on to mental health providers. Therefore capitation, for both mental health and behavioral/lifestyle/health concerns, will likely be an expanding market for psychologists and other behavioral clinicians (Wiggins, 1996).

So, how does capitation work? In a nutshell, capitation involves payment to the provider group "for a package of health services on a prepaid basis, per enrolled, without regard to the actual frequency, extent or kinds of services provided. The amount of a capitated arrangement is calculated on the basis of the expected utilization of services for the covered population" (Yenney & APA, 1994, p. 34). Capitation transfers the majority of the financial risk to the provider rather than the purchaser of services. For example, in one capitated plan to provide family preservation services in a privatized state model of Medicaid, the capitated payment per year per family case to cover all necessary services was about $3500. If the case can be managed with actual costs less than this figure, then the provider gets the difference in profit (or shifts the money to cover unexpected costs on another case).

Providers can conduct in-home intensive family preservation for these difficult-to-treat cases, but (and this is a big but), if the child needs to be removed (e.g., placed in a psychiatric inpatient facility), the provider must pay for the expenses of that placement. Increased expenses of the provider associated with administration, paperwork, and other factors, (and these do usually go up under these plans) must come from the capitated payment. No more money is available for these provider "overhead" expenses. The capitation payment is the total that the system will pay the provider.

An advantage of capitation is that clinicians regain independent control over the type and length of treatment for each covered patient. The clinician may come out ahead financially if the capitation or case rate fee is adequate and he or she sees several patients for only one or two sessions. However, in our experience, this rarely occurs. One of us is aware of a capitation arrangement that currently offers providers $280 per case. However, the managed care company prescreens all potential referrals through an EAP-like process, so those patients requiring only a few sessions (in this case one to six visits) are not referred to an outside provider. Those who are referred require at least several visits to resolve the current problem, thus reducing the clinician's per-visit fee. In several cases, referred patients required hospitalization, the cost of which is taken from the clinician's pocket.

Yenney and the APA's Practice Directorate (1994) recommend that clinicians pursuing capitated contracts seriously consider these issues:

- Calculate estimates of costs using available information on utilization rates, population demographics, and any unique conditions (adjustments must be made on a variety of variables)
- Have a large enough population of covered individuals to spread out the risk
- Control referrals to inpatient and residential settings, as these are the most expensive interventions and costs can exceed the budgeted allocation
- Carefully delineate which services are provided by the clinician under a capitation contract (and which are not)
- Develop protections for radical changes in utilization patterns to stop the losses to the provider
- Include quality of care incentives in addition to the usual emphasis on less expensive services
- Provide information management procedures

Finally, we suggest that capitation plans for the individual clinician are not for the "faint-hearted."

MANAGED CARE AND THE CLINICIAN

We believe that, for a managed care system to be used effectively (for employers, consumers, providers, and even the managed care companies themselves), the consumers (the patients) must be informed and must choose whether restricted care is what they want. Managed care companies make this difficult for the consumer in many cases. We know of one HMO whose member newsletter stated, "[We want] to make it easy for you to get [mental health] services when you need them," and went on to list evaluation, testing, inpatient and outpatient care, and residential treatment as benefits that the member could easily access by simply calling the behavioral intake center. However, this same HMO sent letters to its clinical providers stating that "mental health benefits for most [HMO] members provide short term crisis stabilization therapy," and encouraging *providers* to let the HMO plan members know that extended benefits would not be covered. We think these deceptive practices make it difficult for a consumer to be well-informed about their benefits until they actually need to use them (and find they are not as promised), and they often make the provider look uncooperative from the patient's point of view.

As repeatedly noted, managed care arrangements offer many advantages and disadvantages. The individual clinician must examine all parts of the puzzle in order to find his or her best solution. The difficulty is in maintaining legal, ethical, and competence standards within these changing business conditions.

Practicing outside Managed Care

A woman brought her 14-year-old daughter to a psychologist for evaluation of depression. In the course of the assessment, the psychologist discovered that the child was adopted, her father had died violently and she had witnessed his death 2 years earlier, the father was perceived as her protector from her mother's alternating verbal abusiveness and cold neglect, and the child was failing in her college-prep school, which had been selected by her father. The psychologist was able to spend several sessions interviewing the child and her mother and completing an extensive battery of tests, including intelligence and achievement testing and personality and emotional status testing. During the process, the girl opened up to the psychologist and began making progress, to her mother's delight. The mother also got help for her own depression. The girl and her mother agreed that they wanted the girl to meet with the psychologist weekly and continued this arrangement for 6 months. This was possible only because the mother paid for therapy sessions, which she found useful and valuable, out of her pocket, without limits set by a managed care company. The psychologist did not have to complete managed care forms or "beg" for sessions on behalf of the patient, which likely would not have been judged "medically necessary." The psychologist felt that the ability to see the girl for as long as needed allowed her to develop a significant and supportive relationship, which would not have been possible with the limits imposed by the typical procedures of managed care. The family was quite satisfied with the services received, and the girl's functioning (grades, social involvement, mood) improved measurably.

A psychologist, in private practice with one associate, had a series of negative experiences with managed care and decided to resign from all managed care panels. He carefully planned his new approach to practice and developed a successful business. He estimates his income is 30% from fee-for-service clients, 30% from outside contracts, and 40% from lectures, teaching, and his locally produced television show. His wife runs his office and they have a philosophy of providing the best quality consultation available. He does not discount fees, but provides some pro bono work. This psychologist's income has actually increased since he resigned from all managed care panels.

Developing a successful managed care-free practice requires a dramatic change in thinking about the business of practice: It generally requires what has been called a "paradigm shift." Traditionally, psychologists and other mental health providers have followed on the coattails of medicine in developing independent practices that are dependent on third-party, insurance-based reimbursement. Unfortunately, by following this model, psychology has allowed itself to be subject to the same financial pressures that are also severely affecting the medical care delivery system. As we have seen, this model is increasingly pushing providers into large group practices within hospital-based integrated delivery systems. The insurance industry is attempting to control costs by reducing reimbursements and restricting services more and more. As psychology continues to expend major resources fighting for a slice of the ever-shrinking managed care pie, the opportunities in independent practice continue to diminish. More and more, psychologists are being forced to join large groups, become employees of HMOs, or take other full-employment jobs in order to continue clinical practice. The concept of solo independent practice is fading away like a pleasant dream that vanishes with the demands of the day. In order to work outside of the managed care system, clinicians must refocus their attention on the fundamental marketing issues faced by any small business. The orientation to the medical model will have to be changed, and clinical practice should be recognized for the capitalist enterprise it is. Clinicians will need to start thinking more in terms of running a small business than practicing medicine (or mental health care).

Monetary issues are not the only, or even the primary, consideration of those who eschew managed care. O'Hara (1996) lists several incentives to work outside of the managed care environment:

- Having more time available to pursue the things in life one considers important
- Working in response to one's desire to serve humanity
- Being free and independent in one's practice and business
- Doing what is loved and loving what is done

Although serving the mentally ill is a worthwhile endeavor for clinicians, it is too narrow a focus for those who wish to practice outside managed care. Psychologists, in particular, will need to expand their customer base to include different customers and previously overlooked phenomena. Those who pursue such a practice must look beyond dysfunction and pathology and beyond established medical practices such as prescription privileges. This does not mean that psychologists should not pursue these things, only that they must not limit themselves.

Most psychologists did not learn business principles, marketing, or how to write a business plan in graduate school. Clinicians learned clinical skills such as how to interview, how to make diagnoses, and how to develop a treatment plan. Later, as long as the clinician was employed in a setting where he or she did not need to consider the business aspects of practice or when the climate was such that mental health services were fully reimbursed and there were more patients to be seen than therapy hours available, that mode of thinking was adequate. However, as clinicians seek to establish solo or group practices free from the constraints of managed care, they enter the marketplace as entrepreneurs and businesspersons (and, many times, even within managed care arrangements they function this way). Therefore, the clinician must learn to think outside of the clinical "box." As proposed by one commentator: "What if we start looking for a new, wider customer base and identify potential needs that could benefit from creative new applications of psychological knowledge and skills? What if independent practice begins to mean becoming more customer-focused, rather than product-centered and technique-driven?" (Perrott, 1996, p. 194).

ADVANTAGES TO FEE-FOR-SERVICE CLIENTS

There are several "hidden costs" to consumers associated with managed care practices of which clients may not be aware. When their plan requires referral through either their PCP or an EAP plan, the client must take time off work (or time out of school) to go to the gatekeeper before going to the specialist. This results in increased time (and often money) demands and decreased confidentiality. If the gatekeeper is not familiar with the mental health provider, the referral may be inappropriate, resulting in additional time lost and frustration and further decreasing confidentiality. By either going out of the managed care network or by having other or no coverage for mental health services:

- Clients ensure themselves confidentiality of the highest degree. While many parents do not see lack of confidentiality as a threat to their *child*, the potential problem of securing a government security clearance or policies for health or life insurance later (due to preexisting conditions or high-risk ratings) may be important.
- Clients become partners with the clinician in determining what services are needed and what form of treatment is most suitable to them, rather than having a stranger, and possibly an unqualified one, tell them what to do.

■ If referrals to other mental health providers are needed, the most appropriate provider can be selected without regard to whether that person is on a particular panel.

In addition, one observer noted that "even middle-class clients without insurance will want psychological services, and be willing to pay—if the costs and benefits of therapy (or 'counseling') are presented as similar to other life-enhancing and trouble-preventing activities—orthodontia, car repairs, adult education courses, membership in a fitness club" (O'Hara, 1996, p. 49).

IDENTIFYING AND RECRUITING SELF-PAY (FEE-FOR-SERVICE) CLIENTELE

Because psychologists have been overidentified with medicine, only about 7% of the population would accept therapy, even if it were offered for free. That is, consumers want counseling, not therapy, because "therapy" is too closely associated with the concept of mental illness. By avoiding the mind-set of the medical model and promoting psychologists as specialists who help people with life problems, clinicians can take advantage of this untapped market of people who want and need help. In practical terms, this means marketing services using very different language than is traditionally used in mental health. Rather than advertising that one treats eating disorders, for example, one could talk about helping people who worry too much about their weight or who cannot keep their minds off of food (O'Hara, 1996).

A certain percent of the population will only seek mental health services if those services are covered through their managed care plan. However, another segment is willing to pay for services out-of-pocket if they can choose their preferred clinician and protect their confidentiality. The following ideas may increase the number of fee-for-service clients (McCann, 1996; "Special Report," 1996). Clinicians might:

■ Promote the nonmedical aspects of one's practice, that is, those services that are useful to children and parents who may not have a diagnosable problem. This includes educational, psychological, and possibly spiritual guidance, as opposed to curing an illness.

■ Offer short, educational classes (called "classes" rather than "groups") for free or for a low fee in order to attract clients who want more in-depth help. (We describe these strategies in greater detail later in this chapter). The clinician can call the local newspaper to inquire about listing a low- or no-cost community service. This is potential free advertising.

- Make it known through advertising, such as through the yellow pages or brochures, that the clinician works with a special population, including work exclusively with children, as opposed to all ages. Contacting the local newspaper with offers to help out with reporters' questions about developmental or psychological aspects of children can result in additional free advertising for the clinician; calling often to keep his or her name in the forefront is a good idea. If a tragedy or emotionally charged event occurs in the community, the clinician can offer insights into the situation. However, this will be beneficial only if the clinician has done his or her homework and is thoroughly knowledgeable about the subject. Nothing will harm a practice faster than offering expert advice on things one does not understand.

- Emphasize confidentiality with families. Although many families do not see this as important where their children are involved, the clinician can help them understand the issues involved should they choose to use their managed care plan for their child's mental health services. The wise clinician will discuss the limits of confidentiality with families (parents and children old enough to understand) on the first visit and will ask parents to sign a form indicating their understanding that if they choose to use a third-party payor, the clinician has no control over confidentiality once the information leaves the clinician's office (see Box 3.2 in Chapter 3). It is important for parents to understand that there will most likely be a permanent computer record made that could affect the child's future ability to obtain insurance coverage, gain a security clearance, or even get a specific job later on.

- Educate clients and potential clients about the value of therapy. Using medical cost offset information (see Chapter 7), for example, can help clients and potential clients understand how therapy can help avoid future problems, enhance their parenting skills, enhance their child's performance, and so on. The clinician can keep literature on hand (reprints of articles, summaries, educational brochures) to distribute or show on request. Potential clients can be asked to consider how much it would be worth to them to solve a particular problem or to improve their child's outlook for success in a certain area. The cost of therapy can be compared with the cost of everyday "luxuries" such as a new microwave, the cost of select soccer enrollment, and similar expenditures. In addition, it may be helpful to keep in mind that many other professional services are routinely paid for out-of-pocket, including attorney fees, veterinarian bills, dental care, and accounting services. Although there are no guarantees of success from therapy, the literature provides a great deal of support for specific techniques to treat specific problems. Parents who are unsure can be referred to these articles.

■ Be enthusiastic in "selling" one's services. Too often, psychologists are reluctant to "toot their own horns." Clinicians have a very valuable service to offer. It is important to give potential clients as much information as they need to make the decision to begin therapy. This information might include what the clinician might do to help them or their child with the presenting problem, what length of time it is likely to take, and what the probable costs will be. Parents who attend a class lasting one or two sessions are likely to have more questions and may need some brief individual help, or the class may raise more questions about whether their child does need additional help. The clinician can provide parents with information on cost/benefit and outcome research to encourage them to pursue therapy or assessment if it seems warranted. The clinician can also emphasize the more private and more personalized nature of individual help over classes.

■ Market therapy groups or parent groups to other clinicians as a good way to build the practice. Many psychologists do not offer groups, but have a need for group treatment for specific clients from time to time. If the clinician is seen as a resource for these, the groups offered are more likely to be filled. Clients ought to be referred back to the original source once the group therapy is completed to avoid the perception of "client stealing."

■ Help parents anticipate that it is normal for a child or family to need an additional episode of treatment later when a set of treatments is finished. This information helps parents and children avoid feelings of failure if other problems arise later and keeps the clinician as a resource to be used as needed. Patients can be encouraged to call as needed for future visits or information.

■ Follow up with clients who have finished an episode of treatment by sending out a patient or client satisfaction questionnaire along with a letter asking, "How are you doing?" As detailed in Chapter 4, the survey should ask clients what they liked and did not like about the clinical service and what changes they would suggest (see Box 4.6). This questionnaire serves the dual purpose of demonstrating that the clinician cares about the client and also prompts reflection about whether additional help is needed. When it seems reasonable, many clinicians schedule a 6-month "booster session" to reinforce changes and check on progress. Although a reminder call from the clinician's office may be needed, most clients will return for the check-up visit if one has been scheduled. When recheck appointments are left up to the client to schedule if needed, they are less likely to return.

- Send thank-you notes for referrals and keep in close contact with referral sources. Parents/clients can be asked to sign a release form for this specific purpose, but if they refuse, the clinician can still send a generic thank-you note without mentioning the client by name. This common courtesy can increase referrals. Requesting referral source satisfaction information also communicates concern for quality of care while maintaining contact (see Box 4.7 for an example of a referral source questionnaire). These contacts can identify what the clinician could do to better serve their needs or what additional services they would make use of if they were available. With appropriate client permission, the referral sources can be informed about the outcome of previous referrals. Major referral sources might be called or visited regularly, at least quarterly, and asked about any glitches that may have occurred. Any new services being offered can be described and the clinician can find out if they have specific needs to be met. In addition to primary care physicians, clients can be asked for their permission to contact other referral sources, such as divorce attorneys, ministers, and school counselors. These contacts may not only help the client, but may also contribute to the practice's marketing efforts.

- Do a critical self-evaluation. The clinician can ask colleagues for feedback on relative strengths and weaknesses. Friends can try to schedule an appointment with the clinician, and then find out how much trouble they had with the answering service, the message-taker, arranging billing, and other aspects of the practice. Such seemingly minor details can often make or break a practice.

- Analyze referral patterns and increase marketing efforts toward the actual clientele. If a clinician tends to advertise as a "pain management specialist" but ends up seeing ADHD evaluations primarily, the practice could potentially increase clients by marketing to those referral sources who would make even more ADHD referrals. This does not mean the pain management services should be discontinued, but that the practice may need to be better tailored toward the actual population seen. Or, if the clinician does not want to evaluate or treat ADHD concerns, he or she will need to do a better job of marketing those services actually available to different referral sources (see Box 6.1 for an example of a form for tracking referral patterns).

- Analyze sources of income. Looking at actual income figures may show that managed care contributes little to the bottom line while adding to time and paperwork demands. The clinician may make better use of administrative time by focusing efforts on those sources of income that make up the major portion of the profitability of the practice (see Box 6.2).

BOX 6.1 FORM FOR DATA COLLECTION ON PRACTICE PATTERNS

Practitioner Name: _____ Office:_____

Month:_____ Year: _____

Diagnosis (code + name)	Patient age/ gender	Treatment type	Outcome	# Sessions	Payer	Referral source

How to evaluate above data:

	# Patients	Avg. age	Avg. # sessions	Outcome

Internalizing disorder
(primary diagnosis)

Mood disorders
- Dysthymia
- Major depression
- Bipolar disorder
- Cyclothymia.
- Other

Anxiety and related disorders
- Overanxious or generalized anxiety
- School phobia/refusal
- Separation anxiety
- Specific phobia
- Obsessive-compulsive disorder
- Other

Somatoform disorders
- Somatization disorder
- Pain disorder
- Other

BOX 6.1. (*Continued*)

Externalizing disorders
(primary diagnosis)

Disruptive Behavior Disorders
- ADD/ADHD
- Oppositional Defiant Disorder
- Conduct Disorder
- Other

Tic Disorders
- Tourette's Disorder
- Other

Eating, Sleeping, Elimination
  Disorders
- Enuresis
- Encopresis
- Feeding Disorder
- Anorexia
- Bulimia
- Nightmare Disorder
- Sleep Terror Disorder
- Other sleep disorder
- Other

Adjustment disorders and V-codes
- Adjustment disorder, depressed
- Adjustment disorder, anxiety
- Adjustment disorder, mixed
  anxiety & depression
- Adjustment disorder, conduct
- Adjustment disorder, mixed
  conduct & emotion
- Other

V-codes
- V-codes

Miscellaneous other disorders
- Impulse control disorders
- Problem re: medical condition
- Problem re: abuse
- Gender identity disorders
- Alcohol dependence/abuse
- Other drug dependence/abuse
- Other

BOX 6.2 FORM FOR TRACKING SOURCES OF INCOME

Month _____ Year _____ Practitioner _____

Income source	Intakes	Individual Tx.	Testing hours	Other	Amount billed	Discount	Collected	Due
HMOs (list all plans used this month):								
PPOs: (list all)								
Other managed care:								
Other insurance billed:								
Private pay (full pay patients):								
Contracts:								
Consulting:								
Speaking/writing:								

Teaching: _____

Other: _____

_____

Totals

Total amount collected (_____) ÷ Total amount billed less discounts (_____)

= Percent collected of presumably collectible amount (_____)

Total amount collected from all managed care (_____) ÷ Total amount billed, less discounts (_____)

= Percent of managed care collections (_____)

Total amount collected from other sources (_____) ÷ Total amount billed, less discounts (_____)

= Percent of non-managed care collections (_____)

Total amount collected from one managed care company (_____) ÷ Total amount billed, less discounts (_____)

- Identify an unfilled niche in the community and develop specialized skills to fill that need. Clinicians can develop their strengths and interests and promote their specialization by developing treatment protocols, offering classes, or publishing brief and informative literature. The clinician should visit people who could potentially refer clients in need of one's specialty, and let them know about the approaches one has developed. In doing so, the clinician needs to focus on reimbursable services that are generally not covered by managed care, such as treatment for sleep disorders, parent education classes, services for specific conditions (hearing or vision impairments), psychosocial services for specific medical disorders (diabetes, asthma), and specialized support groups.

- Advertise one's services in a professional manner. Word-of-mouth advertising is important to building and maintaining a practice, but other forms of advertising are also usually needed. These might include business cards, brochures, newsletters, and regular advertising in affordable media outlets. The clinician should recognize that the more familiar the public is with the clinician and his or her practice, the more likely they will choose that clinician when seeking services.

- Focus on developing services that are paid for by the recipient, such as divorce and custody mediation, consultation to schools and daycare centers, specialized support groups, child abuse assessment, and similar services. People sometimes forget that most other professional services are not reimbursed by some third party. Individuals pay out-of-pocket for attorney, accountant, veterinarian, and other professional services mostly without question. Psychologists can begin to refocus their business efforts to mirror those of other professions not plagued by managed care.

- Develop a professional support group of clinicians with whom discussions can be held regarding cases, treatment outcome, and brainstorming about future business opportunities and practice development. We suggest clinicians schedule regular meetings and *limit complaints about managed care*. The focus in these meetings should be productive and solution-generating rather than complaining.

FINANCING AND PAYMENT OPTIONS

Contrary to popular belief, price is often not that important to consumers in choosing which product to buy or which service to use. *Value* is of considerably greater importance. The temptation to lower prices because business is slow or in order to compete with managed care pricing should be carefully considered. People are willing to pay for quality and service, so instead of reducing fees, clinicians might emphasize the quality and service offered by their practice. The goal should be to deliver more value than the other guy (including the managed care system).

"Segmented pricing" refers to the practice of offering the same product at different price levels, based on some factor such as volume of business, cash payment, and so on (Levinson & Godin, 1994). Some segmented pricing is illegal, so it is important to check with an attorney familiar with health care law and/or with one's state licensing board or professional association before engaging in such practices. If the type of segmented pricing the clinician is considering is legal, the most important consideration is that the pricing rules appear fair to those paying the higher prices and that lower prices are available to anyone who meets the criteria for discounted fees. For example, if a clinician offers a 10% discount to all clients who pay cash, those who chose to pay with a credit card may feel that the convenience of their payment plan outweighs the value of the discount. However, that client may also decide that it would be worth it to pay cash in order to save 10%, and the clinician should be willing to accept this discounted fee since it meets the same criteria. (Discounts for cash may violate the practice's agreement with the credit card company, however, so the clinician must check this.)

Simplified pricing (set fees for defined services) may be a good option for some clinicians. It can help in marketing because the predictable cost of a specific service can be discussed in advance and therefore make the actual cost known to the consumer (or referral source) prior to purchase (Levinson & Godin, 1994). For example, the clinician might offer an ADHD evaluation consisting of interviews with specific informants, a classroom observation, parent and teacher questionnaires, and a feedback session for a set fee. An additional fee could be specified for inclusion of intellectual and educational achievement testing when those are not provided by the school. In such a simplified pricing arrangement, the pediatrician, school counselor, or parent knows in advance what will be provided at what cost, and may choose to call other clinicians to compare prices. It is often helpful for potential clients to know in advance what the full cost of service will be so they can make such comparisons in personal budgeting and evaluate whether they can afford to purchase that service.

Following are some payment and financing options to consider in order to increase fee-for-service referrals (depending on the specific legal arrangements of the clinical practice):

- Offer a discount for cash payments at the time of service. This arrangement avoids the extra expense of having to file on a client's insurance, the expense of credit cards, and the possibility of insufficient funds checks being returned. Clinicians offer from 10–20% discounts over their regular fees for cash payments.

■ Offer credit card payments. This arrangement is convenient for most clients who may not keep enough in their checking account to cover their weekly therapy appointment or for the considerably larger expense of psychological testing. If they have difficulty paying the entire balance, their credit card will generally allow them to pay it out over a period of time of their choosing and the clinician will not be left waiting months for payment.

■ Remember that a psychologist is not a bank. Clinicians should not make a habit of carrying patient balances. Instead, they can offer credit card payment options and allow the clients to arrange their own payment plan through the credit card company. It is important to note that a lot of dissatisfaction, litigation, and complaints to state boards result from payment disagreements. If clients pay for services as they are rendered and are informed in advance of financial arrangements, the likelihood of these problems is greatly reduced.

In establishing fee payment arrangements, it is usually illegal to offer different fee structures based solely on the availability of insurance. The clinician must be certain that any financing arrangements cannot be construed as being based on the availability of insurance. Some clinicians offer a "discount" by writing off the client's copayment. In most cases, while practicing within managed care, it is a violation of the managed care contract to discount or fail to collect a copayment. Clinicians should avoid engaging in this practice unless the managed care company has confirmed that it is not a violation of the contract. Again, while working with a managed care contract, most managed care companies make payments based on the clinician's "usual and customary charge," so if certain discounts are offered outside managed care, then a managed care company fee reimbursement may also be reduced. Discounts for cash payment are not likely to fall under this rubric, but other discounts, such as "professional courtesy," may.

As previously noted, psychologists are not bankers, and it is unreasonable to expect a clinician to carry large balances without interest for clients. However, at times, the clinician may make exceptions and agree to allow a client to pay out a balance over time. If the clinician chooses to do this, it is important to get the financial arrangements stated in writing, with amounts due and payment due dates. Any penalties for late payments should be mentioned in the contract along with what the clinician will do in the case of nonpayment. Many clinicians have found that once clients finish treatment it becomes easier for them to ignore an outstanding balance, especially if they do not anticipate seeing the clinician again. A clinician should fully inform all clients regarding the practice's policies on payments, insufficient funds checks, and penalties for late cancellations and failure to show for appointments. The client should be given the information in writing as well as verbally and should be asked to sign a consent form indicating that they have received the information and agree to the provisions (see Box 6.3). This form can protect the clinician to some degree in the case of a complaint to the licensing board or a lawsuit from an unhappy client.

GOALS/STANDARDS FOR PRACTICE AS A BUSINESS SETTING

When a clinician enters the independent practice of psychology (or other mental health field), he or she opens a small business. During the 1980s, psychologists did not need to worry much about the business aspects of their independent practices because their business was based exclusively on providing assessment and therapy to people outside of hospitals, community mental health clinics, and university teaching clinics where there were seemingly plenty of available consumers. Other psychologists were employed by mental health clinics and hospitals and were not independent businesspersons. However, in uncritically following the medical model of practice, psychologists followed a beguiling, yet treacherous, path into reliance on the insurance industry for reimbursement. As we have seen in recent years, this path is now squeezing more and more "service" out of providers for less and less reimbursement.

To have a successful independent practice today, the clinician must think of the practice as a small business and of himself or herself as a small business-person. This reorientation involves several steps, including writing a mission statement, writing a business plan, and establishing professional relationships with a banker, attorney, and accountant, among others. It involves marketing a "product" (service) and seeking new markets and new products, all while conscientiously following the ethical guidelines of the clinician's profession.

The first step in starting a new business (or revamping an established one) is to develop an idea and then create one or more products or services based on that idea. Next, the clinician-businessperson must find probable markets for the services/products (see the next section, "Marketing"). Discussing these ideas with a trusted friend or colleague can help the clinician ascertain if the idea has potential as well as determine other variations that could be added to the product/service list or marketing plan.

Once the idea has been well considered, a business plan should be developed formally. The business plan should include business structure, financing,

BOX 6.3 SAMPLE CONTRACT FOR A
FINANCING AGREEMENT

_____ (Responsible party) agrees to pay the balance due for professional services provided by _____ (Provider's name) in accordance with the following:

Principal amount due is $ _____

Payments of $ _____ are due on the (_____ and) _____ day of the month, beginning on ___/___/___.

Payments will be considered late if not received in the business office, located at _____, by the _____ day of the month.

Late payments will be charged a penalty of $ _____ per late payment. Late payment penalties are due by the next payment due date.

Interest charges of _____% of the remaining balance will be incurred if a payment is not received within _____ days of the due date, or _____.

If payments are chronically late (late for more than 3 months), the full balance, with accrued interest, will become due on the _____ day after the third late payment.

Unpaid accounts or remaining balances not paid on time will be turned over to the District Attorney's office or to a collection agency on the _____ day after a payment is missed.

I have read and fully understand the terms of this agreement. I agree to abide by and intend to fulfill this contract.

_____   _____
(Signature of responsible party)   (Printed name)

_____
(Address)

_____   _____
(Home phone/work/other phone)   (Social Security Number)

_____
(Driver's license number/state issued)

marketing plans, and an operational schedule (Perrott, 1996). There are a number of resources available to help the new entrepreneur. If the clinician is unsure how to write a business plan, it will be necessary to either learn how or hire someone who knows how. The Service Corps of Retired Executives (SCORE), a service of the U.S. Small Business Administration, offers many services to persons opening or planning to open small businesses. They can be found in the telephone book business pages in most major cities, and some chapters have Internet sites (search the Web through the Yahoo search engine by the key word "Retired Executives" or, for example, find the Cincinnati chapter at: www.score.chapter34.org/index.htm). Business-oriented associations and clubs (Chamber of Commerce, Rotary, Business Women's Association) can also be good resources and good marketing venues.

In reexamining the concept of independent clinical practice, one must consider three major changes: an expanded customer base, additional professional services, and a market-based business process (Perrott, 1996). First, the clinician should consider expanding the customer base, as the traditional customer base for psychologists is the small percentage of people with mental illness, behavioral or developmental disorders, or significant problems of daily living who were willing to seek professional help and who had some means of paying for that help. Given the low rates of utilization of professional services, approximately 90% of the population can be considered a potentially untapped market if there is a product or service that the clinician can offer.

The second change, adding professional services, requires clinicians to develop and offer services other than psychotherapy. Psychologists are well trained in using scientific methods, research-based knowledge, and professional skills to address a vast array of human problems and potential. Roberts (1994, 1996) reported on several creative "model programs" of mental health service delivery that developed new ways of addressing both familiar and new problems when there were no apparent solutions readily available. This type of creative approach to the concerns of children and families can be translated into new markets and new products and services.

Third, developing market-based business practices, requires the clinician to think as a small businessperson in terms of developing a business plan, marketing, and other aspects of business that have not been adequately addressed by most independent practitioners in the past. We will look at marketing in depth in the following section.

MARKETING

Starting or revising a business to sell professional services today requires more sophisticated marketing strategies than ever before. The clinician who enters private practice must deal with all the aspects of business faced by any other retailer or service provider, including cash flow, marketing, balance sheets, research and development, business ethics, and human resource allocation. In today's health care market, there is a greater need to differentiate one's services from those of others who are targeting the same market and providing similar services. Perrott (1996) recommends that psychologists position themselves as "customer-intimate" market leaders. That concept means expanding the customer base to include not only those with dysfunction and pathology, but also that other large percent of the population that could benefit from psychological services adapted to different customer needs. The characteristics of these new services, according to Perrott, would include the following:

- Customers would be active participants, rather than passive recipients
- Services would be solution-generating, rather than problem-centered
- Procedures would aim to increase customer knowledge and skills, rather than focus on deficits and deficiencies
- Relationships between customers and change agents would be interdependent, rather than hierarchical. (p. 195)

Once these ideas have developed into potential services with some form and substance, they must be incorporated into a viable marketing plan. An idea with no means of expression is not a basis for a business. Successful businesses can provide guidance in this area, but following the medical model will not necessarily be useful. A comprehensive marketing plan must include a mission statement, target population, and marketing budget. The clinician will also need to develop solutions to the "four Ps of marketing" (product/service, place, price, and promotion) based on the idea (service, product) to be marketed.

The mission statement is simply a sentence describing the purpose of the service or product. The mission statement helps define the direction of the business. Levinson (1993) recommends condensing the idea for one's business to seven sentences, and then to seven words or less. Wall, Solum, and Sobol (1992) recommend a "vision statement," which includes a glossary to define terms used in the vision statement and a set of guiding principles, in addition to the basic mission statement. This instrument helps everyone associated with the business practice work in the same direction and helps the owner/clinician to stay focused on the target goal. As the clinician specifies what the goals of the marketing plan will be, the target population is narrowed and defined. Finding ways to present and position the clinician's service requires ingenuity, creativity, and boldness. The marketing budget will further refine the marketing plan. It is important for the clinician to remember that marketing is necessary, not just desirable, to have a successful business, and too little attention or time devoted to marketing will result in less business. Many clinicians find the idea of marketing off-putting, but when those ideas are examined, they generally reveal distorted concepts of what marketing really involves. We have found that Jay Conrad Levinson's book, *Guerilla Marketing* (1993), includes some very practical and useful marketing ideas for clinicians hoping to practice outside of managed care. He states, "Every component that helps you sell what you are selling is part of the marketing process. No detail is too insignificant to be included. The more you realize that, the better your marketing will be" (p. 9).

Marketing is the way people learn about the practice, but it is also the way people remember to make referrals to a particular clinician. If a clinician does not market his or her practice, referrals are very likely to slow significantly. As a rule of thumb, a clinician should plan to spend 20% of his or her working hours doing marketing. Although this may sound like an extraordinary amount of time, marketing, as defined here, can include some income-producing work. For example, if the clinician offers a parenting class, each parent in attendance should receive a handout that includes the clinician's name and phone number and at least one business card (stapled to the handout). Giving two business cards to each person allows the person to keep one and give the other to a referral. If clinician attends a clinic 1 day a month, each patient and each physician should receive a business card at every visit. Even if a doctor was given a card last month, the clinician should give one again this month because this may be the month that the physician will need to make a referral. Any handouts developed by a clinician should be on that individual's (or group's) letterhead or at least have the clinician's name, address, and phone number on the first page.

It is reasonable for clinicians to expect to do some free work in the interest of marketing. For example, the child-oriented clinician could give a lunchtime talk to a pediatric group (nurses included) on a topic of their interest (psychological evaluations, depression in children, pain management). It is not necessary to provide lunch, because it will add to the marketing cost and may not be included in the marketing budget. Presenting at "grand rounds," if the clinician practices in a locale with a teaching hospital, is a productive way to be seen by a large group of potential referral sources. Presentations to professional groups such as nurses and physicians may help them with institutional inservice training requirements (and possibly continuing education credits needed for registration/licensure). Talks on managing the adolescent patient, for example, may enhance the participants' understanding, but may also generate referrals when the adolescent patient is not so easily managed.

Additionally, the clinician should keep in mind that physicians (and others) may need help in the mechanisms of making a referral. Often, they feel that it will be insulting to their patients to receive a mental health referral (it usually is not), or they do not know which patients would be appropriate to refer for services. The clinician can assure them that it is okay for the physician to call if they are unsure or that, for example, the clinician does not mind seeing a child who does not meet DSM-IV criteria for a diagnosis or who may only be having minor adjustment problems.

The clinician can focus on the functional aspects of the problem—if the physician perceives a problem in the child's functioning, the clinician might be able to help remediate the problem even if the child does not meet the criteria for a diagnosis. The clinician should emphasize that this is often a fairly short-term and relatively inexpensive process (not the "three times a week on the couch for 5 years" that many physicians associate with "psychotherapy"). Such concerns may present opportunities for the clinician to develop new products or services and may offer untapped markets (classes for parents of children undergoing chemotherapy, teacher training in classroom management of problem behaviors or reintegration of the child with a chronic illness).

In developing other markets/products, clinicians can offer to provide direct or indirect services (assessments, inservice training, parent workshops), consultation, or other services that are lacking or inadequate in the schools. Even providing some services on a pro-bono basis can increase the likelihood of additional referrals to the practice or requests for consultation in the future. Educating potential referral sources about how the clinician approaches a problem can also make them more comfortable making the referral. If they cannot imagine how anyone could help a preschooler control his anger when the child barely talks, they may feel foolish making the referral. When the referral source understands that the clinician might help the parents with some behavior modification techniques that will result in the child expressing anger more appropriately, they may then more enthusiastically make that referral. One cannot assume that even pediatricians know what psychologists do, because they may not. It would be appropriate for the clinician to ask if they would like to hear about how the clinician approaches the problems about which they are concerned.

Business Cards

Every piece of paper that has the clinician's or business's name on it reflects on the quality of one's practice. Therefore, it is important to have business cards printed on high-quality paper that stands out from other cards. It may be worthwhile to hire a designer to develop stationery products (business cards, letterhead, brochures) that reflect the uniqueness of the clinician's business and tell as much about the clinician as possible in a small space. A business card that lists one's name, degree, and "psychologist" tells little to the prospective patient or referral source. One that indicates a specialty, such as "clinical child psychology," and indicates specialized services ("specializing in assessment and treatment of eating disorders") can help increase the number of appropriate referrals and can be a ready source of information for someone seeking a referral for their patient with anorexia, for example. Using the back side of the business card for additional information about the clinician or the practice is a relatively inexpensive way to provide a larger amount of useful information that is easily kept at hand (Levinson & Godin, 1994). The potential referral source who receives such a card can file it, refer to it once the details of conversations have faded, or offer it to a patient who has heard five other names of possible clinicians in the past week. Business cards should be distributed as widely as possible. These are an inexpensive and easy form of marketing that can have a large impact on business.

Practice Information Brochures

Brochures describing the clinical practice and the credentials of the clinician should also be printed on quality paper and should be professionally written, designed, and produced. Levinson and Godin (1994) suggest either a three-fold brochure on preprinted forms or a low-cost four-color flier folded into a booklet. There are several sources of good quality, preprinted papers available (see Levinson & Grodin, 1994, for resources). Brochures should contain a great deal of detailed information about the clinician's services. They should be distributed selectively, such as to potential clients who call for information, school administrators who may need a consultant for a specific need, or others who might need the additional detail about one's practice that is included in a brochure.

Parent Education Groups and Classes

Conducting brief, targeted workshops is an exceptional way to market a clinician's availability and competence in the community. Advertisement in newspapers, on public access television, in daycare centers, and through after-school programs can bring the clinician's name and expertise to the forefront. Parents can be charged a modest fee for participating. For example, Dr. Carolyn Schroeder and colleagues in Chapel Hill Pediatrics conduct a number of workshops in the evening and at lunch hours. The evening classes involve no more than 20 parents of children of similar ages and cover such topics as Living with Toddlers, The Preschooler, The School-Age Child, and The Challenging Adolescent. For the three school-age child programs, the clinicians present didactic information, answer questions, and give handouts on Setting Realistic Expectations; Developing Cooperation; Chores, Homework, and Relationships; and Discipline without Shouting or Threatening. The Schroeder group's "lunch and learn" programs include Tips on Limit Setting, Toileting Training, and Building

Self-Esteem, among others. Schroeder and Gordon (1991) provide additional information on these services.

Community Presentations

The clinician can make presentations to civic groups such as Kiwanis, Optimists, Rotary, Junior League, and others. The talks need to have a theme of general interest and some strong points of position (e.g., sex and violence on television, helping children be children rather than miniature adults). The presentations should not just focus on children's mental health problems and the clinician's services (i.e., these talks must not look overtly like advertisements). In addition to talking to nurses and physicians, as mentioned earlier, child management issues might be presented to the local dental society using examples of poor techniques observed in other practices. Talks to parent–teacher organizations might focus on parents' needs to manage a busy lifestyle while still being available for their children, stress management, time management, and how parents can make sense out of all the parenting advice on television and in print. In all the public presentations in the community, the clinician will need to individualize the topic and content to the interests of the audience and have material ready to distribute about his or her practice

Community Consultation

Many clinicians have found community consultation to be a positive aspect of a primary care-based practice. For example, through a primary care pediatric office, Schroeder and Gordon (1991) coordinate all the community agencies involved with abused children. This collaboration grew from an educational focus into defined roles for the various players. The mental health professionals became case managers and developed contracts to provide group treatment for sexually abused children. Their service has now expanded to include school-based services, including sex education and abuse prevention at all levels. The psychologists, in collaboration with school personnel, developed the program, trained the teachers, and informed parents. This has further expanded into psychologists providing training to court-appointed Guardians Ad Litem, judges, district attorneys, the state department of social services, the rape crisis center, the YMCA, daycare centers, and other community agencies. One can see, through this example, how identifying a niche market, developing an idea to approach that market, and being willing to have the idea expand could result in a significant portion of one's work coming from outside managed care. It is assuredly more difficult for the solo practitioner to work out such an elaborate plan independently. However, this example clearly demonstrates the value of collaboration and community consultation.

Child Guidance Brochures

The clinician can provide printed brochures and pamphlets to give developmental and clinical information useful to the parent, extend the clinician's reach, and provide a marketing tool for the practice. The pamphlets often get handed around and may generate further referrals. The clinician needs to ensure that the brochures are based on the best available information and are consistent with the clinician's therapeutic practices. These are related to the treatment protocol handouts described in Chapter 4, but include more general information useful to parents (and less specific treatment prescriptions). Dr. Edward Christophersen and his colleagues at Children's Mercy Hospital in Kansas City, who are behavioral pediatric psychologists, have developed a large number of protocols and handouts to give parents for a variety of child-rearing problems. Christophersen (1994) has collected these in one resource with explanations for their use by the practitioner. These handouts include such topics as:

- Discipline for Toddlers: Time-Out
- Toilet Training Resistance
- Managing Excessive Crying
- Peer Interaction Skills
- Separation Anxiety
- Redirecting Your Child's Activities
- Teaching Self-Quieting Skills for Toddlers
- Grounding as a Method of Discipline
- Behavior Problems in Public Places
- Attention-Deficit Hyperactivity Disorder

Drs. Carolyn Schroeder and Betty Gordon, private practitioners in Chapel Hill, North Carolina, have prepared a "Parent Series" of handouts on a variety of topics. Stamped with their practice logo (name, address, telephone number), these one- to four-page printed pamphlets deal with the following topics:

- Negative Behavior: How to Manage It
- Fears: Dealing with Your Child's Irrational Anxieties
- Toilet Training
- The New Baby: Helping Older Children Adjust
- Managing Children's Anxieties

- Sexuality: Helping Children Understand and Appreciate Their Bodies
- Divorce: Helping Your Child Adjust
- Sleep: Helping Older Children Adjust
- Habits: Thumbsucking, Pacifiers, Nailbiting and Tics

Dr. Russell Barkley (1991) developed an ADHD fact sheet for clinicians to give out to parents and teachers. Dr. Nicholas Long and his colleagues at the Department of Pediatrics of the University of Arkansas for Medical Sciences wrote a series of one- to four-page handouts as part of the Parenting Research and Education Program. These flyers include such topics as:

- Time-Out as a Discipline Technique
- Teaching Children to Follow Directions
- Stress Management for Parents
- Children's Self-Esteem
- Managing Mealtime Behavior
- Children's Development: Fifteen to Eighteen Months
- Children's Development: Eighteen to Twenty-four Months
- Children's Development: Two to Three Years
- Helping Children Cope with Stress
- Parental Communication
- Sibling Rivalry among Older Children
- Handling Slow Dressers

In Figures 6.1 and 6.2, we present two sample handouts from this group to illustrate how these child guidance brochures can be useful.

The clinician may also find it useful to develop handouts on events as they arise. Drs. Connie Fournier and William Rae, psychologists in an HMO at Scott & White Clinic in Texas in the early 1990s, developed several circulars during the Desert Storm/Gulf Crisis for children and families affected by the military assignments and actions. One-page briefing sheets were distributed on:

- Emotional Support Strategies for Parents
- Emotional Support Strategies for Schools
- Grief Reactions in Children
- Telling Children about Death (for School Personnel).

As can be seen, these independently developed handouts have a commonality of topics derived from frequently asked-for information from child clinicians. Although not likely to resolve major psychological difficulties, these protocols can be useful adjuncts, while publicizing the clinician's practice for larger

Parenting Research Education Program

BITING

Biting is a behavior that is not uncommon among young children. The reasons why children bite other people differ from child to child.

It is quite natural for children around one year of age to bite their parents or anyone else who happens to be within reach. Most often in this age group, children bite to reduce the pressure on their sensitive gums due to teething.

True biting, not due to teething, can become a problem with children between 18 and 30 months of age. Children at this age are often unaware of the pain that biting causes to other children and to adults.

Although it is common for children to bite others while playing, this type of behavior warrants immediate action. Not only is biting extremely painful for children who are bitten, it often leads to more fighting within the play group. Biters also run the risk of becoming unpopular with their playmates.

Young children often bite in response to frustration, anger, or excitement. Thus, it is important for parents and caretakers to be aware of what situations lead to biting behaviors. Such knowledge may help parents better understand the causes of biting behavior.

What Can Be Done?

Biting is not something that has to be endured until children are old enough to "know better." There are many steps that can be taken to both prevent and solve biting problems.

Prevention

•**Set Limits.** To prevent biting from occurring, parents and caretakers should set limits before young children play together. Rules should be simple, like taking turns and sharing. Parents and caretakers should consistently enforce these rules.

•**Catch children being good.** Parents and caretakers should compliment children for getting along. Complimenting children will serve as a reward for good behavior. It will provide recognition to children who behave instead of to those who misbehave.

•**Supervise play closely.** Parents and caretakers should pay attention to what is going on in the play group. They should intervene before conflicts get out of hand. Structuring play periods may cut down on the opportunities that lead to biting.

•**Watch what you teach.** Parents and caretakers who use yelling, spanking, or any aggressive behavior as a form of discipline for children run the risk of teaching children that aggressive behavior is acceptable in certain situations, especially in solving conflicts. Adults who hit, yell, and/or throw things when they are mad are teaching their children to be aggressive when they are mad.

Intervention

•**Identify times when biting occurs.** Parents and caretakers should observe times

Department of Pediatrics
University of Arkansas for Medical Sciences
Arkansas Children's Hospital

Page 1

Figure 6.1. Parenting research and education program: biting.

and situations when children resort to biting. They should use this information to change or avoid these situations. For example, if children bite whenever they play in a large play group, steps should be taken to limit the number of children in the group. Or, if children bite whenever they are with a specific playmate, steps should be taken to separate the two children during play time. If a pattern to the biting behavior is detected, the situations that lead to the biting behavior, if possible, should be avoided. It may be necessary for parents and caretakers to simplify play times, to make play groups smaller, and to make play periods shorter.

•*Use brief time outs*. Parents and caretakers should use a brief reprimand, such as, "No biting. Biting hurts. Time out." They should then place the children who bite in time-out. These children should be allowed to return to the play group after they are quiet and under control. Parents or caretakers should then provide positive attention, showing children who bite that there are better ways to communicate and be noticed.

•*Provide alternatives to biting*. Parents and caretakers should tell children what they can do instead of biting. For example, "Instead of biting when you're mad, just walk away." Or, "Instead of biting when you're mad, ask the teacher for help." Children should then be asked to repeat the alternatives back.

•*Focus attention on the child who was bitten*. Parents and caretakers should give all the toys, fuss, and attention to the bitten child. If children bite for attention, or to get a reaction from adults, they will soon learn that there are better ways to be noticed. If, for example, one child bites another in a dispute over a toy, the toy should be given to the bitten child. This will teach biters that biting will not bring about the desired result.

•*Seek professional help for persistent biting*. If biting continues to be a chronic problem despite repeated attempts to intervene, professional help may be necessary to clarify the reasons for biting and to eliminate the behavior.

What Not To Do

Biting should **not** be ignored in the hope that it will quickly go away. In most cases, it will not. No matter how frustrated parents become in their attempts to eliminate biting in children, biting children back to teach them a lesson is **NEVER** recommended. If this sends any message at all it is that adults hurt people, too. In most cases, very young children are unlikely to make any connection between the hurt they feel from being bitten, and the hurt they have caused by biting.

Things To Remember

In most cases biters cease biting as their language skills increase. As language skills improve, children become able to use words to express frustration and anger. This usually occurs around the age of three. With firmness and consistency in confronting and dealing with biting behavior, most biters get the message and quickly stop biting.

Finally, a bite that breaks the skin can cause an infection. If the skin is broken, it is important to wash the injury thoroughly with soap and water, and then apply a sterile dressing and secure it with adhesive tape. A doctor should look at the wound as soon as possible.

Figure 6.1. (*Continued*)

Parenting Research Education Program

TEACHING CHILDREN TO FOLLOW DIRECTIONS

One of the most challenging tasks that parents often face is teaching their children to follow directions. It becomes frustrating for the whole family when parents have to repeatedly give their children the same directions ("Pick up your toys"). The recommendations below can be of assistance in teaching children to follow parental directions the first time they are given.

•Parents should avoid giving their children a direction unless they are prepared to enforce it. If parents do not enforce their directions, then children learn that their parents don't mean what they say.

•Parents should always get their children's attention before giving a direction. Parents should avoid yelling directions from another room.

•Parents should avoid phrasing directions as questions (for example, don't say "Justin, would you like to pick up your toys now?").

•Parents should avoid giving vague directions such as "Be good," or "Be careful." There may be significant differences between how the parent and child interpret vague directions such as "being good." Parents should make their directions clear and specific.

•Parents should try to give directions that tell children what to do instead of what not to do. For example, it is better to say, "Stay by my side," than "Don't run away."

•Parents should praise their children as soon as they have begun to follow the direction. Parents don't need to wait until the task is completed to offer praise.

•When the task is complete, parents should let their children know they appreciate their compliance.

•If children do not start to follow a direction within ten seconds, parents should put them in time-out immediately.

•Parents should avoid giving their children repeated warnings. Children can learn to follow directions after one or no warning just as easily as they can learn to follow directions after five or six warnings.

•After the time-out is complete, parents should repeat the direction to their children. If they do not start to follow the direction, time-out should be used again. This process should be repeated until children comply with the direction.

Department of Pediatrics
University of Arkansas for Medical Sciences
Arkansas Children's Hospital

Figure 6.2. Parenting research and education program: teaching children to follow directions.

problems likely to be covered under a health care plan or for parents self-paying for treatment. Often, just copying another practice's brochures will not be as useful as the clinician's own effort. In cases where the ethics of this practice have been challenged, adding the clinician's name to another's brochure or newspaper column has been seen to imply authorship and deemed unethical. Developing and printing these brochures will initially cost some money, but may have pay-off later in increased referrals. Additionally, philanthropic organizations may wish to co-invest in brochures if they are consistent with their purposes, and credit for the support is given.

Newsletters

Publishing and distributing a newsletter can make the clinician's business practice a source of information as well as service, and it keeps the name "up front" in the minds of potential clients and referral sources. An effective newsletter must be targeted and filled with short facts and "bullets" of information. It is better for the newsletter to cover a wide variety of topics briefly than to bore readers with too much detail or by going on too long. Newsletters should be short—not more than a few pages—and educational. Most importantly, a newsletter should be distributed on a regular, dependable schedule, not just every now and then or when one has some free time. Before embarking on a newsletter, the clinician should spend some time deciding on the specific goals for the newsletter. It should have a clear purpose that will direct all the material that appears inside. As with brochures and business cards, a newsletter must have a professional look and feel that reflects the quality of the practice.

Mailing Lists

Keeping a mailing list is a good way to increase one's exposure. Whenever anyone calls the office, whether to get information or to schedule an appointment, the person's name and address should be added to the mailing list (with the caller's permission). The clinician can offer to send a brochure to a caller as a good way to add an address to the list. More sophisticated mailing lists can include information about the individual, such as ages of children, types of concerns (divorce, school problems), whether the caller scheduled an appointment, or other important information. If the clinical practice has a specialty focus, it will be easier to know what sorts of information are needed on the mailing list. The list can then be used to send targeted mailings regarding upcoming classes or about new services. Then, once a class has been held, more names might be added to the list.

Internet Marketing

Marketing through the Internet is a recent phenomenon, with as yet unproven effectiveness. However, the general impression seems to be that group practices, and many independent practitioners, will have their own Web sites in the near future. Clinicians can be "linked" to other sites, such as their local area or state psychological associations or other relevant hot links. As with other forms of marketing, it is important to focus on quality and to design (or have designed) an outstanding Web site. Following are some things to consider in designing a Web site:

- Have limited graphics (graphics can take a long time to download)
- Make the site visually attractive by using vibrant colors and an easy-to-view format
- Offer consumer-friendly information, such as might be included in a newsletter
- Include information on contacting the group or clinician by phone

Some Web sites include on-line intake forms and E-mail access to clinicians. We recommend that clinicians use caution and avoid ethical problems by using on-line access to *receive* information only. We do not support providing counseling or therapy via E-mail.

Other Web sites offer psychological assessment via therapist-produced questionnaires. Again, we caution that this could violate ethical principles of psychologists and that clinicians must be cognizant of the guidelines for test development and of potential copyright violations if the clinician offers tests on-line that have been produced by others.

ACCESSIBILITY

Being accessible is one of the key ingredients to a successful business. The clinician simply cannot provide services without being accessible. This means the clinical practice should have convenient hours, but also easy parking, for example. The clinician should also be available to do school and home visits and should always return phone calls as soon as reasonably possible, at least during the same day. Other considerations that make a clinician more accessible include:

- Accepting credit cards

- Having a good system for answering the phone and taking messages (a major problem in primary care settings)
- Having handicapped accessible office and building

Accessibility is as diverse a concept as marketing, and no less important.

DIVERSIFYING REFERRAL SOURCES

The clinician may need to expand the range of referral sources by thinking "beyond the box." The days of waiting passively for patients to appear in the clinician's office are fairly well gone. Children and adolescents often are in situations such as schools, medical settings, summer programs, and youth groups where adults see the need for psychological assistance. Some of these settings come with built-in reimbursement possibilities, others will be fee-for-service in the parental self-pay circumstances. The following are potential referral sources for marketing efforts (suggestions are elaborated upon from those offered by the APA Practice Directorate, 1996):

- School districts (assessments, consultation on specific problems): Traditionally trained school psychologists may have all they can handle with their own specified duties. Clinical child clinicians capable of assessing and treating more serious emotional disorders are often needed. For example, one of us (MCR) was consulted in setting up a therapeutic classroom for elementary school children with DSM-IV diagnoses. The special education teachers and school psychologists were already overcommitted to the pupils needing their services, so outside consultation was necessary.
- Private schools and church-based schools: These schools often do not have access to services that are available through the public schools and are frequently in need of psychologists for inservice staff training and for referrals and consultation.
- Community agencies (women's shelters, rape crisis, suicide prevention, grief centers): Children are frequently ignored in settings serving adults. Education about the need for services for children appearing in these community agencies and services the clinican can offer might open possibilities for consultation and treatment.
- Police departments, judges, juvenile justice agencies (giving talks, consultations, expert witness testimony, court-appointed evaluations): There is an increased recognition of (and new money available for) the need for psychological services in these domains.

- Businesses and large employers (giving talks, contracting through EAP): Giving talks to local businesses can generate referrals and can potentially pay well. The clinician can develop two or three topic areas with handouts and can then be ready with a year's (or more) worth of presentations. Parenting talks and "divorce impact on children" talks are popular topics.

- Daycare centers: The clinician can develop consultative relationships with daycare centers for inservice training, child management, and direct line referrals.

- Churches: Increasingly churches are engaging in outreach services to members of their congregation and others in the community (e.g., homeless shelters, drug and alcohol support, violence prevention programs, grief groups, divorce recovery classes, parenting classes). The clinician can assist in the development of these services and receive financial support for the professional services. For example, one of us (MCR) worked as a paid consultant for a group home run financially and administratively by a religious organization (this setting had been developed by the active efforts of another psychologist who later transferred the consultantship).

- Civic groups: Many philanthropic and service organizations have strong commitments to programs for youth. The clinician can develop concepts for interventions that fulfill their missions in a targeted program. For example, the clinician could seek funding that could be relatively modest and short-term, or larger and longer. The list of potential service clubs would be too long to detail here, but the clinician might move beyond the more obvious ones (e.g., Kiwanis, Rotary, Optimist, Sertoma, Junior League) to the multitude of study groups, etc. in each community.

- Divorce mediation (mediation services, custody evaluations): The clinician might circulate a position/assessment approach about custody to local attorneys that may generate more consultation and referrals. One of us (MCR) coauthored a paper published in a psychology and law journal on divorce and custody issues. He and his coauthor distributed copies to all the lawyers handling divorces in the community; they were inundated with calls and referrals (including many of the lawyers' personal custody situations).

- Self-help groups: The clinician can provide talks and information or serve as an expert consultant for such groups as ADD/LD, and CHADD and hospital-based groups for chronic illness such as diabetes and asthma.

■ Hospitals: The clinician may offer expert consultation to the volunteer or hospital auxiliary in improving preadmission familiarization tours for children and parents, outpatient clinics, assessments, treatment protocols, and consultation.

Although the clinician is not likely to be able to use *all* of these suggestions, this list of expanded referral sources and settings for potential income is suggestive of how the clinician may diversity and think expansively about possibilities.

Contracting

If a clinician is associated with a larger group of psychologists or mental health providers, he or she may be able to negotiate directly with employers for mental health/behavioral health contracts. If so, an attorney should review all contracts, and a certified public accountant should be engaged to evaluate the financial aspects of the contract. We strongly urge that clinicians approach capitated contracts with caution, as the financial risk falls directly on the provider should utilization be underestimated. This outcome can be financially devastating. The advantages of direct contracting (not capitated) relationships is that third-party administrators and UR entities are more limited in their impact on one's practice. Such contracts should emphasize wellness, health outcomes, and appropriate risk-sharing. The clinician must first identify a large enough group of providers who are diverse enough to provide all the mental health coverage needed or have access to other services that may be required only occasionally. The group should be balanced in terms of expertise and specialties.

If the clinician is a solo practitioner or in a small group, he or she may not be able to contract directly with employers. However, it might still be possible to provide services on a limited basis, such as by offering to give lectures to parents ("selecting a child care facility," "separation anxiety in preschoolers," "is your child's trantrumming a problem?"). This approach is particularly likely to succeed in a company that has wellness programs and values employees' mental health as helpful to the company overall. For example, the business may be willing to contract with the clinician to do a monthly "Lunch & Learn" seminar or an after work lecture series. They may also provide the space to do a series of meetings on a particular topic, with either the company or the employees paying the fee. The clinician may need to educate employers about the value of providing such benefits in order to open the door for one's services (see Chapter 7). If a solo practitioner is considering offering such classes as a marketing tool, it would be wise to determine what insurance plan the employees use and whether the target audience is likely to seek out independent (self-paid) consultation with the psychologist. For example, a lecture to a group of hourly, minimum wage workers will have far less marketing potential than a lecture to middle or upper managers (although it might be a good activity, the focus here is on keeping the clinician in business). The benefits of providing "free" seminars to management would thus likely outweigh other presentations.

WORKING IN PRIMARY CARE

Setting up a clinical practice in a primary care setting leads to diversification of the practice in many ways. Acting as "health psychologist" on a primary care team leads to opportunities for work with treatment adherence and response as well as health promotion, even though these "problems" may not be reimbursed by insurance. Primary care physicians today do not have the time, always, to build the kind of relationships with patients that will allow them to identify stressors and psychosocial factors that affect their patients (not to mention the fact that patients often change primary care doctors annually as their managed care plan is changed by their employer). A psychologist in the primary care office can address those psychosocial factors that interfere with compliance or limit effectiveness of medical treatment (Hersch, 1995). Cummings (1995) adds that the psychologist can fill the void left by the familiar general practitioner who heard all the family's upsets and distresses and helped them cope through each one. He proposes that the psychologist can provide multiple episodes of brief therapy throughout the life span.

Other advantages of working in a primary care setting include: (1) early identification of mental illnesses or developmental disabilities that require longer or more intensive traditional psychological treatment, (2) increased physician and nurse awareness of psychosocial factors that affect physical health, and (3) increased patient comfort in accessing psychological services within the familiar primary care environment (Hersch, 1995). Our experience has been that primary care physicians welcome psychologists as colleagues, not as subordinates or "physician-extenders," and that their awareness of psychosocial issues and treatments increases with additional exposure to the psychologist in their office (Drotar, 1995; Roberts, 1986).

In primary care, there are a variety of models of service delivery that may be different from traditional independent practice (Roberts & Wright, 1982). The psychologist may be part of a team or may be called on to provide a quick screening and brief interview as needed while the patient is in the office for a medical appointment. The psychologist may offer services (classes, groups, or consultation) related to normal aspects of life such as the birth of the first child, how to toilet train, concerns about daycare center selection, and so on. None of these are likely to be covered by insurance benefits but are nonetheless appreciated enough that parents are often willing to pay for them.

Psychologists can also affiliate with other health care professionals to enhance their services. For example, associations with dentists to help with phobic patients or overly anxious parents, or with speech pathologists or occupational therapists to work with the behavioral aspects of feeding problems are potential opportunities to expand one's practice. When the clinician is knowledgeable about various disease processes and medical conditions, his or her input regarding the psychological aspects of illness will be appreciated. Just as the clinician is happy to answer the physician's questions about behavior and mental health, we have found that most physicians are generally happy to explain medical illnesses or physical structures to psychologists.

Working with sick children as a consultant in a hospital setting is another way to diversify the clinician's practice. The role of the psychologist in both helping the child with compliance, coping, and stress related to his or her illness and helping the family become part of the treatment team in order to adapt to the child's illness and emerging health is quite valuable (Hersch, 1995). The specialty field of pediatric psychology and child health psychology is described more fully in other resources (Peterson & Harbeck, 1988; Roberts, 1986, 1995; Roberts & Walker, 1989a).

Scientific Bases for Clinical Practice in Managed Care

A clinical child psychologist was denied membership on a managed care panel ostensibly because the company wanted mostly generalists who would see anybody referred to them. This clinician appealed the decision in a meeting with the provider relations director using a briefing letter describing the benefits of specialty training in services to children, adolescents, and families. She provided additional information on "medical costs offset" when brief psychotherapeutic treatments for children were employed (techniques previously demonstrated to be in this clinician's armamentarium). The clinician was eventually added to the panel and referred a number of clients utilizing her special skills.

In this chapter we want to provide clinical research information useful to the clinician in responding to managed care. This information includes as much justification as possible for the things that clinicians do in their work, such as the empirical support for child psychotherapeutic interventions, cost savings when psychological services are provided, acceptability of psychological treatments, quality of care demonstrations, and documenting what the clinician does in practice. We think it is important and pragmatic for the clinician to have this information ready at hand. Perhaps this issue was best articulated by a *Psychotherapy* article:

> Psychologists must learn to market effectively to third-party payers, hospitals, and consumers to show what we can offer. In today's competitive health care market, we must be able to demonstrate specifically where psychological services are unique and provide better treatment than medicine or other mental health professions. (Ludwigsen & Enright, 1988, p. 427)

In other words, we need to know what we can do and document it. We also need to know and remember where most of the quality research on mental health services and outcomes comes from. Psychology, straddling both science and practice, is in the best position to understand and utilize the massive amount of research and apply it to practice. Once, listening to a talk radio station while driving, one of us was astounded to hear a physician claim that psychologists could not employ biofeedback for psychophysiological disorders because these were "medical procedures" to be used only by "medical doctors." A quick-thinking psychologist called in asking who had conducted the research supporting the efficacy of biofeedback for the disorders for which he claimed it worked and asking where the research had been published. Although not backing away from his exclusionary claim to biofeedback, the physician finally acknowledged that most of the founding work had been done by psychologists and published in psychology journals. Similarly, clinicians need to know and remember the foundations of training that set the discipline apart from others. In this chapter, we provide the basics of the research for a quick reference by the clinician. Follow-up to the referenced articles will provide more detail.

DO PSYCHOLOGICAL TREATMENTS WORK?

The clinical professions are often faced with challenges to justify the types of interventions employed in practice. The efficacy, effectiveness, and cost benefits of therapeutic interventions have long been issues for academic researchers and practicing psychologists. We provide information here to assist clinicians in supporting the variety of therapeutic modalities utilized in clinical child psychology practice. Many commentators have noted that much of clinical child and adolescent psychology practice employs techniques not as firmly planted in empirical support as the field might need or the managed care corporations might demand. Notably, however, the number and range of empirically supported *medical* practices are more limited (see Lipsey & Wilson, 1993; Parloff, 1984).

When many of today's practicing clinicians were trained, they were often required to read the child psychotherapy outcome studies by Levitt (1957, 1963). His narrative review of the studies completed at those times essentially replicated the findings of Hans Eysenck in 1952 in which he found that psychotherapy was no better than spontaneous remission of symptoms. These reports were fairly discouraging for us as therapy novitiates because they basically concluded that traditional therapy with children did not result in any substantial therapeutic gain over what happened to children who had been placed on waiting lists or baseline control lists. As a result, many in the profession sought to establish effective treatments through behavioral and cognitive behavioral modalities.

Later narrative and qualitative reviews have taken a more positive view of psychotherapy outcomes for children. The development of meta-analysis has also been a major boon to interpreting the variety of statistics resulting from the multitude of treatment outcome studies. Rather than conducting a qualitative (and often subjective) review of treatment outcome, the meta-analytic approach quantitatively combines all reviewed studies to produce a mean effect size statistic. The larger the average effect, one concludes, the more effective the intervention was. Three meta-analyses have been reported for psychological treatment of problems of children and adolescents (Casey & Berman, 1985; Kazdin, Bass, Ayers, & Rodgers, 1990; Weisz & Weiss, 1993; Weisz, Weiss, Alicke, & Klotz, 1987). The following conclusions can be drawn from these significant works:

- Psychologically treated children were functioning better after treatment than were the control group children, aggregating across all studies and forms of therapy. (Generally, these results match those regarding psychotherapy with adults [Smith & Glass, 1977].)
- The results support behavioral interventions over nonbehavioral approaches (although some reports indicated no solid evidence of one type of treatment as more effective than any other).

Notwithstanding any limitations of the studies included or the meta-analysis methodology, there is considerable consistency in these conclusions across the meta-analyses: *Psychotherapy with children is effective* (or, in the careful conclusions of science: *Psychological treatment results in effects exceeding any change resulting from not receiving treatment*). More focused meta-analytic studies have examined particular types of interventions such as family therapy (Hazelrigg, Cooper, & Borduin, 1987), cognitive behavior interventions (Durlak, Fuhrman, & Lampman, 1991), and child and adolescent behavior therapy (Allen, Tarnowski, Simonian, Elliott, & Drabman, 1991). One study conducted a meta-analysis on 302 meta-analytic studies (Lipsey & Wilson, 1993). It concluded that any limitations do not diminish the conclusion that "well-developed psychological, educational, and behavioral treatment is generally efficacious" (p. 1181). Their analysis revealed which interventions have stronger effects for certain problems.

In an interesting and very significant analysis, Lipsey and Wilson (1993) compared the relative findings of therapeutic outcomes of psychotherapy to those of medicine. While hardly reassuring for all of us utilizing medical care, these comparisons indicate that psychological treatments are at least equally or more provably effective than medical interventions. Mental health clinicians, therefore, need not humble themselves before a medical care "gold standard"—because it does not exist. One might argue that the burden of proof is on medicine to demonstrate efficacy of its interventions before reimbursement rather than relying on clinical lore in support. Getting the word out on psychological foundations remains an important task. Clinical researchers in psychology have been appropriately cautious and critical as scientists, yet the strength of this discipline's interventions demonstrate considerable practical worth.

In November 1995, *Consumer Reports* published results of a mammoth reader survey of mental health care use, asking the question, "Does therapy work?" This study concluded that "therapy for mental health problems can have a substantial effect" (Consumers Union, 1995, p. 735). Martin Seligman, a psychological consultant to *Consumer Reports* for this survey, noted that "patients whose length of therapy or choice of therapist was limited by insurance or managed care did worse" (Seligman, 1995, p. 965). Granted, most of the approximately 7000 respondents were describing their own adult experiences with psychotherapy, although parents seeking help for their children's problems might have been included. While it does not meet many standards of psychological outcome research and cannot conclusively demonstrate once and for all time that psychotherapy works, clinicians might appreciate that it serves as some welcome and useful information added to the scientific foundations of clinical practice.

In several surveys, what clinicians presently report doing in their practices is often not what the researchers have examined in therapy outcome studies (e.g., Kazdin, 1993; Shirk & Russell, 1992). While some have used this discrepancy to urge researchers to evaluate what clinicians actually do, others have argued that practicing clinicians also need to practice in ways that the research literature actually supports as effective.

What should the clinician take from all the studies? First, there is consistent evidence that psychological therapies with children do work. Second, some approaches are more therapeutic than others for certain identified problems. Certainly, despite the limitations and criticisms, the clinician can point to the strength and consistency of the positive outcomes of child psychotherapy. Moving clinical practice closer to the empirically supported modalities clearly puts the clinician in a better position of claiming to managed care organizations and other consumers that these positive effects of therapeutic interventions deserve reimbursement to the fullest extent possible.

"FITTING THE PAN TO THE HAM"

Much of the work in psychotherapy outcomes and clinical utility has been guided by the often-quoted axiom about the need to determine which treatments work with what problems under which circumstances (Paul, 1967). That is, treatment decision making must be evaluated in terms of "(a) what therapy, (b) under what conditions,

(c) for which children, (d) at what developmental level, (e) with which disorders, (f) under what environmental conditions, (g) with which concomitant parental, familial, environmental, or systems interventions" (Saxe et al., 1988, p. 803). This formal articulation is often recognized by clinicians as the need to individualize treatment plans for the child and family depending on a well-thought-out diagnosis. Unfortunately, many of the managed care plans diminish the diagnostic and assessment phase by cutting payments for this professional activity. Then, a "cookie-cutter" approach to treatment is fostered by managed care protocols restricting intervention modalities or applying rigid limits to sessions.

Increasingly, clinicians, no matter from what theoretical camp of psychotherapy, accept that no single treatment approach is going to be effective for all problems presenting to the child clinician. Indeed, with over 230 published forms of child therapy identified by Alan Kazdin (1988), clinicians have rejected the "uniformity myth," that is, the assumption that all problems can and should be treated by the same therapeutic approach (Shirk & Phillips, 1991). Whereas it has taken clinical psychology some time to adopt an approach that centers on the client's needs and problems rather than centering on allegiance to a theoretical camp, it has taken managed care entities only a brief time to move the field backwards—such that all clients receiving a particular diagnosis are to be treated the same.

Dr. William Rae (1987), writing in a slightly different context, called this process "fitting the pan to the ham." He cited one of his graduate professors as describing the story of his family cooking a Christmas ham. Asked why she cut substantial pieces off the ends of the ham, a search of family memories revealed that every generation had done it dating back to when the family had only a small pan to cook in. Rae went on to suggest that, "Like the mother cooking the ham, children's health care professionals often problem solve in the same way they always have done in the past, with similarly wasteful results" (p. 216). Similarly, Ron Fox (1995), a leading advocate for private practice in psychology, and past president of the APA, noted that studies of practice patterns reveal that clinicians rely on those treatments that they prefer, rather than treatments that are individualized for patient needs. Additionally, two noted child psychotherapy commentators have asserted that the selection of treatment strategies should be based on the legitimate potential for effecting change, not on the clinician's loyalty to a particular treatment method or theory (Shirk & Phillips, 1991). In this process, clinicians need to evaluate the effectiveness of various treatment approaches and to use empirical research to inform and guide their diagnostic and intervention practices. This will result in more competent practice, and interventions will more likely be reimbursed under managed care systems.

The strongly demonstrated efficacy of behavioral interventions, whether by meta-analysis or other clinical research, creates a conflict with the surveys of practice patterns and allegiance to treatments deriving from psychodynamic and psychoanalytic traditions. This conflict may also be evident in dissatisfaction with the constraints often placed by managed care on psychological services. Mental health services in HMOs tend to be for fairly specific problems that are most amenable to brief, targeted interventions (Bittker & Idzorek, 1978; Brady & Krizay, 1985; Finney, Riley, & Cataldo, 1991). The focus on rapid symptom reduction and behavioral management techniques appears most effective for many of the presenting problems of childhood (e.g., toileting problems, behavioral noncompliance, sleep disorders, psychosomatic complaints). For example, in one behaviorally oriented consultation service within an HMO, clinicians found that about 76% of the parents reported improvement following treatment, with a high degree of parent satisfaction with the services (Finney et al., 1991). Indeed, several professionals have suggested that behavioral therapists may have an easier time adjusting to managed care dictates than will psychodynamically oriented ones (e.g., Armenti, 1993). Accordingly, writing in *Behavior Therapy*, Mash and Hunley (1993) suggested:

> [R]elative to other therapies, cognitive and behavior approaches have a tradition of being the most sensitive to economic concerns of accountability and cost-effectiveness. As such, there is a natural fit between the interests of managed care organizations for cost-efficient interventions with demonstrable outcomes and behavior therapists' long-standing commitment to empirically tested, time limited treatments that yield appreciable changes apparent to the client, the clinician, and others in the client's life. (p. 68)

These authors go on to note "the frequent statements made by proponents of managed care that behaviorally trained clinicians are best suited to act as providers in managed care systems (e.g., Armenti, 1991; Broskowski, 1991)" (p. 68). Apparently recognizing the inherent behavioral orientation of managed care, various professionals have suggested "behaviorizing" the clinician's language, but without changing any aspect of actual practice or theoretical orientation. Thus, psychodynamic concepts are translated behaviorally such that "feelings expression" becomes "management of affect/mood," "calming influences" becomes "stress management," and "psychotherapy" becomes "problem-focused intervention." The ethics and legality of such translations are questionable. In some cases, the techniques supported in other theoretical camps are essentially the same as those practiced by behavior or cognitive-behavior therapists. But in other cases, this renaming is not only inaccurate but downright deceitful.

The scientist-practitioners in the discipline must continue to evaluate empirically the process and outcome of psychological interventions. Practicing clinicians, however, must remain appraised of the growing literature and shape their practice patterns within these newly emerging parameters. We believe strongly that the scientific evidence, as best as can be provided, rather than intuition or belief, will secure psychology's place within the health care field whether in managed care arrangements or larger systems. To this end, fortunately, some help is available to the clinician who is seeking established interventions for the varieties of problems presenting to the practice. For example, other books in this *Clinical Child Psychology Library* series provide clinician-oriented information on a pragmatic approach to anxiety and phobic disorders (Silverman & Kurtines, 1996), parent-child interaction therapy (Hembree-Kigin & McNeil, 1995), and assessment and treatment of sexual abuse (Gordon & Schroeder, 1995). Additionally, the newsletter of the Division of Clinical Psychology, *The Clinical Psychologist*, has been publishing articles in a series entitled "Empirically Validated Psychological Treatments" (Task Force, 1995). To date, only a few treatments for children's problems have been noted: parent management training for oppositional and conduct problem children (Feldman & Kazdin, 1995) and behavioral treatment of enuresis (Houts, 1996). Presumably those techniques having been reviewed and found empirically supported would stand a better chance of receiving approval for managed care reimbursement. This remains to be seen, however. Other interventions, not making it onto the list, may suffer total exclusion from the reimbursable protocols. The clinician is always well advised to stay current with these professional developments. Fortunately for the practicing clinician, many other interventions for disorders manifested by children, adolescents, and families have received empirical support.

MEDICAL COST OFFSETS FOR TREATMENT OF CHILDREN AND FAMILIES

Clinicians have been frustrated by the lack of easily interpreted facts in a centralized location providing information on treatment effectiveness and its value in managed health care systems. Once, in preparing for arguing to preserve reimbursement for psychological services in Medicaid plans at the state level, for example, one of us needed hurriedly to search the clinical and research literature for examples of cost savings from mental health services. Of the literature summaries that exist, most are oriented toward adult psychological treatment (e.g., Friedman, Sobel, Myers, Caudill, & Benson, 1995; Groth-Marnat & Edkins, 1996; Sobel, 1994). We cannot provide a full analysis of how psychological services for children and families can save money for HMOs, but we do set out here some basic information for the clinician.

One particular form of cost savings for HMOs potentially comes from providing some services that reduce the members' use of medical services. This savings is called "medical offset." In particular, while providing psychological/behavioral treatments may cost a certain amount to the HMOs, if an enrollee so served has a lessened need to seek more expensive medical services, the HMO achieves a cost offset from the psychological component. Thus, rather than add to costs, psychologists can help lower them overall. The premise of cost savings from psychological services derives from the recognition that approximately 60% of all physician visits have no diagnosable medical disorder (Cummings & Follette, 1968). Therefore, mental health principles become more salient. Studies conducted in the early stages of HMOs have supported that medical costs are offset by psychological services (Cummings & Follette, 1968; Mumford, Schlesinger, Glass, Patrick, & Cuerdon, 1984).

The "offset" effect has also been demonstrated for child psychological services. One of the early studies including child patients examined the impact of psychological evaluation and treatment on such variables as medical outpatient units, number of pharmaceutical prescriptions, presenting medical problems, and the relationship of psychological diagnosis and medical services utilization (Rosen & Wiens, 1979). A matched control group of patients permitted comparisons. Psychological services were provided through a medical psychology outpatient clinic for a range of diagnoses receiving a variety of evaluations and services. Rosen and Wiens found several important results:

- Patients receiving psychological services decreased their medical usage by 41%.
- Patients receiving psychological services also significantly reduced their number of prescriptions and the number of presenting medical problems.
- Psychiatric inpatient hospitalizations (very expensive services) decreased by 35% following the psychological referral.

Thus, the provision of appropriate psychological evaluation and treatment significantly reduced the medical utilization of patients experiencing psychological distress and problems.

A similar study was conducted in a neighborhood clinic for children and adolescents in a diverse cultural and ethnic population (Graves & Hastrup, 1981). The psychological interventions took a problem-solving approach utilizing behavioral and family systems theories. This study found that:

- Clinic patients receiving psychological treatments significantly reduced their medical clinic visits from a mean of 5.8 in the previous year to a mean of 3.7 in the year following psychological contact. (The control group did not show such a decrease.)

- A matched control group (having similar psychological distress, but untreated) slightly increased their visits from a mean of 4.7 to a mean of 6.1 visits.
- After treatment, patients displayed medical utilization rates not different from a random control group in the clinic.
- Mental health interventions by psychologists reduced medical utilization rates by 36%.

Recent studies have found similar results in that the offset effect was obtained by psychological services and consultation on pediatric outpatient use (Finney et al., 1991). A Behavioral Pediatrics Service was set up as a psychological consultation service with the Columbia Medical Plan, an HMO in Columbia, Maryland. After screening for appropriateness of referral, the children and their families received brief targeted therapy (essentially behaviorally based) for behavior and emotional problems, including problems in school, psychosomatic complaints, toileting issues, and behavioral concerns. Parenting instruction was provided in behavior management techniques of time-out and reinforcement. Contingency contracting was frequently used. These clinical researchers found that:

- Intervention resulted in reports by 76% of the parents that the referral problem was resolved or improved (corresponding to 80% of the therapists' ratings).
- Satisfaction with the services was reported in 82% of the parents (very satisfied and satisfied).
- Objective assessment indicated the therapists' interventions were effective, reducing both externalizing and internalizing referral problems.
- Psychological treatments significantly reduced medical encounters from the pretreatment (8.75 visits per person year) to the posttreatment (6.43 visits per person year) levels.

Thus, these clinical researchers found that the provision of brief, problem-focused interventions to children presenting with behavior, psychosocial, and toileting problems significantly reduced the use of medical care services in contrast to previous use rates. In addition, the clinical researchers reported that even with the addition of the specialized psychological consultation for behavior problems, the children's total use of HMO services did not increase.

A second study in this setting examined how psychological treatment affects children with recurrent abdominal pain who are excessive users of more expensive medical care (Cataldo, Finney, Lemanek, Katz, & Fuqua, 1989). In this therapy outcome study, children with recurrent abdominal pain were treated in the pediatric psychology consultation service based in the HMO. Interventions were individualized for each child utilizing behavioral principles (e.g., self-monitoring, dietary modifications, limited reinforcement of pain symptoms, relaxation training). Their results found that:

■ Psychology treatment sessions were effective (2.5 visits on average with additional phone calls).
■ Parent and therapist ratings indicated 81% problem resolution or improvement and reductions in school absences.
■ After receiving psychological treatment, the children showed significant declines in the number of medical visits per month compared to their pretreatment levels and to a comparison control group.

Thus, the multifaceted but brief interventions were not only effective, but also resulted in lower usage of medical services in the HMO. In a strong cautionary note, however, Fraser (1996) argued that "the rush to sell psychology through broadly predicted medical offsets may be starting to backfire on even the best of managed behavioral health care groups" (p. 335). He suggests that "all that glitters may not always be gold" (p. 336).

What do findings of medical offset studies suggest for the clinician vis-à-vis managed care entities? Several studies have found that the children who use more medical services, in general, tend to have more psychosocial problems (e.g., Diaz et al., 1986). Indeed, the mental health problems of an HMO enrollee may be the critical issue in excessive (and expensive) medical care utilization. Given this fact of more costly services, we suggest that clinicians or groups of clinicians seeking to break into the managed care market may wish to challenge the managed care organizations to a test, with an evaluation component attached.

The clinician can ask the health care corporation to identify those families that are the highest users of medical services in the HMOs. Then, by studying the characteristics of the use and needs of the frequent users, the clinician can identify those, for example, whose problems are not catastrophic medical conditions. The clinician can look for those families and children whose accessing of medical services appears highly mediated by psychosocial concerns. Then, the clinician can offer to the managed care organization to treat some of these high medical care users in carefully planned behavioral health interventions for a higher than typical fee for psychological services. The clinician should keep careful records to document that the cost of the psychological intervention is less than the previous use of more expensive medical services. By documenting medical offsets in one's own practice, the managed care case managers, given their orientation to cost savings, should come to value the clinician's efforts at long-term savings to the corporation.

We should note that some research in HMOs has found that the cost savings may not be evident for some time (Hankin, Starfield, Steinwachs, Benson, Livingston, & Katz, 1984) because the families have to learn to shift their service requirements to the psychologist rather than physicians. Additionally, a recent study indicated that treatment of psychosocial problems through mental health interventions decreased patients' medical costs only for the older children. This decrease resulted from fewer non-mental health specialty care visits; that is, the primary care visits were not reduced (Kelleher & Starfield, 1990). Small-scale studies can be conducted by the clinician to demonstrate the value of psychological interventions. For example, Pfander and Seagull (1992) analyzed the impact of in-hospital psychological consultation to the emergency room in a general hospital for adolescent suicide attempts.

We caution, however, that one should not offer mental health services in a managed care organization only with a goal of cutting costs. While saving money for the company is one business goal, providing relief from psychological distress and behavioral problems is an equally worthwhile goal. Many of the cost savings generated by managed care financing arrangements come from reduced numbers and amounts of services or reductions in the "excess utilization" of inpatient and outpatient services. It is unclear whether any utilization is simply considered inappropriate and unnecessary, or just an individual's use that was over the average use. We think it is a "no-brainer" to state that offering psychological services in an HMO arrangement will lead to use of those services. Of course, people will be attracted to services they need. Not providing those types of necessary services at a high level of quality is not only immoral, in our view, but also short-sighted in light of the medical offset findings described here. Managed care programs may try to minimize availability of mental health services in a variety of ways. However, these programs are likely to end up losing money in the long run because children with psychological problems and their families will access other services (viz, medical) in an attempt to find the needed help.

TREATMENT ACCEPTABILITY FINDINGS

One way of describing the value of mental health approaches to managed care decision-makers derives from the literature on "treatment acceptability." Envisioned as one method of assessing social validity of psychological/behavioral therapy, acceptability of treatment includes attitudes and judgments of clients, professionals, and the public about the procedures used in psychological treatments that are considered reasonably useful and appropriate for the presenting problem and characteristics of the client. Perceived acceptability of a treatment is thought to be associated with adherence to and motivation for treatment, reduced attrition during treatment, and enhanced therapeutic gains. (Client satisfaction, as noted in the next section, is typically a measure of perceptions and attitudes during and after psychological treatment, whereas acceptability is a measure of attitudes toward therapy in general and prior to treatment.)

A fairly substantial literature base has developed distinguishing acceptability of various alternative treatments for certain types of presenting problems (e.g., Kazdin, French, & Sherick, 1981). With interventions for problems of children and families, there are a number of potential views regarding treatment acceptability, besides those of the managed care decision-makers, including children and their parents, school professionals, and medical care providers. We quote here from one integrative and comprehensive review on the key findings relevant to supporting psychological services within managed care environments:

> Acceptable interventions (defined as those achieving mean scores greater than the midpoint on the particular acceptability measure) include positive reinforcement, positive practice, differential reinforcement, and response cost. Interventions rated as unacceptable across studies include corporal punishment, shock, and paradoxical interventions. Receiving mixed reviews are time out, overcorrection, ignoring, token systems, stimulus control, medication, and reprimands. As a general rule, interventions designed to increase behavior where it is deficient in quantity have been rated as more acceptable than interventions designed to reduce inappropriate or excessive behavior....One exception to this general rule is response cost. This procedure is consistently rated as an acceptable strategy to decrease negative behavior. (Calvert & Johnston, 1990, p. 65)

Several forms of common psychological interventions have not been evaluated sufficiently or at all in terms of treatment acceptability. For example, play therapy, family therapy, social skills enhancement, and many cognitive behavior techniques have received little attention (Calvert & Johnston, 1990). Because the focus of treatment acceptability has been on many of the behaviorally oriented techniques, the clinician may need to develop some measures of acceptance of particular interventions usually employed in one's practice.

CONSUMER SATISFACTION FINDINGS

As noted in Chapter 4, one form of outcome measurement is the use of consumer/patient satisfaction questionnaires. This form of information can be useful for a clinician's understanding of his or her own practice and for documentation to a managed care organization. Many clinical practices have institutionalized consumer satisfaction as a matter of routine. In this section, we will review some examples of this outcome measurement. Consumer satisfaction questionnaires and telephone interviews, for example, were utilized from the start-up of the pediatric psychology programs at Chapel Hill Pediatrics, North Carolina, by Dr. Caroline Schroeder. A series of publications, remarkable for full-time private practice, has emerged detailing all aspects of their practice (e.g., Schroeder, 1996; Schroeder & Gordon, 1991; Schroeder, Gordon, Kanoy, & Routh, 1983). As outlined in these publications, the information gathered and analyzed helped focus the clinicians' attention toward improving services, offering new programs, and altering elements rated less favorably by the respondents.

Particularly useful in the information systematically collected by the Chapel Hill Pediatric Psychology group are the parent feedback ratings for treatment effectiveness and service evaluation. Specifically, the evaluation of the innovative "Come-in/Call-in" service found that, across areas of concern, an average of 91.3% of those using the service reported it as good, and only a small percentage reported the service as bad or mixed. Evaluation of the treatments offered for specific areas of concern (e.g., the referral problems) indicated highly favorable perceptions of services for problems in sleep, negative behaviors, and sibling/peer relationships. Lower evaluative ratings were obtained for treatments of developmental delays. This group also obtained parents' ratings of effectiveness of individual aspects of the treatment advice given for specific problems. For instance, for negative behaviors, the advice "focus more on positive behaviors by giving more praise and special time" and "reward appropriate behavior with stars or charts" was rated at averages of 4.78 and 4.57, respectively (out of a possible 5.00). The advice "ignore inappropriate behavior" was rated at a mean of 3.58. Similar evaluations of specific advice or treatment interventions were gathered for interventions for toileting problems, sleep disorders, sibling/peer interactions, developmental delays, and personality/emotional problems.

Parent consumer satisfaction ratings of mental health services have been infrequently assessed in managed care environments (particularly HMOs). In one report of a behaviorally oriented clinical service, 95.7% of the parents reported via telephone interviews that they liked the treatment recommendations made by the clinicians in a behavioral psychology clinic (Charlop, Parrish, Fenton, & Cataldo, 1987). Overall, 100% of the respondents thought the suggestions "made sense," 80% reported the clinicians' recommendations were not difficult to follow, and 82.4% thought the treatment received was beneficial to their children. The parents' global evaluation of satisfaction with the services provided revealed that 89.5% were either satisfied or very satisfied, with only 1.3% reporting being extremely dissatisfied. A later report of parent satisfaction with this behavioral pediatric service found that, after termination from treatment, 93% of the parents whose children were seen in the clinic reported being very satisfied, satisfied, or somewhat satisfied (Finney et al., 1991).

As an illustration of a consumer satisfaction evaluation of a special program, Dr. William Pelham conducted a multilevel evaluation of a summer therapeutic camp for children diagnosed with attention-deficit disorders (see Pelham et al., 1996). These clinical researchers asked parents for ratings of their child's overall improvement (Pelham & Hoza, 1996). They found that 96% of the respondents reported their children as "somewhat, much, or very much improved," whereas only 1% reported the child as "unchanged." Specific variables of behavior were also assessed with ratings of improvement at levels of "somewhat, much, or very much":

- Following home rules   95%
- Adult-directed defiance   95%
- Cooperativeness   92%
- Responsibility   89%
- Self-esteem   84%
- Social skills   84%
- Happiness   58%

Of the parent respondents, 82% and 93%, respectively, indicated "Yes definitely" to the questions, "Would you send your child again?" and "Would you recommend the program to other parents?" Over 80% of the parents perceived the treatment program as very beneficial for their children and themselves. Over 95% reported that their children liked the summer camp. Although these results are encouraging and, indeed, flattering for a intensive and comprehensive clinical intervention such as that found in these summer camps, the information also permits the clinician to focus on certain aspects of the experience or clinical activities for improvement (Pelham & Hoza, 1996).

REFERRAL SOURCE SATISFACTION

Assessing satisfaction about services from those who referred a client to the clinician is an important additional element to measure. However, such referral source inquiry has rarely been conducted. Fortunately, some reports do exist to indicate its worth in documenting quality of service and for enhancing professional relationships with those who recommended the clinician's practice. For example, a 26-item questionnaire was used to assess the perceptions of professionals (viz, physicians, nurses, and social workers) regarding pediatric psychology consultation and liaison services for medical inpatients in a children's hospital (Olson, Holden, Friedman, Faust, Kenning, & Mason, 1988; Olson & Netherton, 1996). These referral sources were queried about numerous aspects of the consultation/liaison service. Specifically, the satisfaction items utilized 1 to 5 Likert-type scales. Through this questionnaire, these clinicians found:

- Satisfaction with overall services was rated   3.6
- Usefulness of feedback was rated   3.7
- Perceived effectiveness of services was rated   3.5
- The likelihood of making future referrals was rated   4.3
- The negative impact on patient care resulting from   4.3
-    a discontinuation of pediatric psychology services was rated

These mean ratings provide information for the clinicians about areas of satisfaction and areas in need of improvement. The respondents also provided a very worthwhile evaluation about the negative impact of potential cutbacks in services. Thus, even in the absence of any other data about treatment effectiveness, the respondents reported that mental health services of this type are essential to patient care in its totality. A similar evaluation was conducted at the University of Florida Health Sciences Center of sources of referrals to the Pediatric Psychology Service (Rodrigue et al., 1995). Overall satisfaction with clinical psychology services was fairly high (mean ratings of 4.0 on a 5-point scale), and similar ratings were obtained for usefulness of feedback and recommendations, and written feedback. The referring professionals also reported a high likelihood of making future referrals to these clinicians. A lower rate of referral source satisfaction (3.3) was obtained for follow-up after the child patient was discharged from the hospital. Such documentation of referral source satisfaction is likely important for future contracts with managed care companies.

While most consumer satisfaction ratings are completed by adults (parents), a few reports demonstrate child and adolescent patients' evaluations of their own experiences in mental health treatment. For example, Garland and Besinger (1996) described an interview and questionnaire used to assess adolescents' satisfaction with three outpatient settings: a school-based clinic, a psychiatric clinic, and a clinic for maltreated youth. These clinical researchers obtained a wealth of qualitative and quantitative information. They noted that general satisfaction was high. Key factors in achieving positive ratings appeared to be the type and accessibility of services matched to needs, the quality of the personal relationship with the health care providers, and the perceived effectiveness of the interventions. Garland and Besinger concluded that "adolescents are quite capable of discussing their expectations, concerns, and satisfaction with mental health services" (p. 372).

A word of caution, however, is necessary. Client or customer satisfaction is subject to manipulation and misinterpretation. Several managed care organizations now require the collection of consumer satisfaction measures, either in addition to or in place of outcome evaluation. There are several obvious problems with consumer satisfaction measures used exclusively to evaluate psychotherapy. First, the process of seeking therapy and finding someone to talk to is often a relief in itself. Therefore, patients whose benefits are limited to only a few sessions may report an increased sense of well-being and high satisfaction with treatment but may not have made any or much measurable progress on specific problems (Howard et al., 1993). Second, customer satisfaction is based on numerous factors that may be totally unrelated to the actual process of therapy, such as availability and cost of parking, how the phone is answered, and friendliness of the business office staff (Morrison, 1996).

Morrison (1996) suggested that customer satisfaction can be increased by training patients about what to expect before treatment begins. When such "role preparation" is done, there are fewer dropouts, and satisfaction ratings increase. In addition, the clinician can work to develop a collaborative relationship with patients. This is good marketing, and increases the probability of positive outcomes. Morrison (1996) reported that if a patient understands his or her role in therapy, he or she is more likely to comply and do his or her part rather than expecting the clinician to do all the work.

Customer satisfaction is the result of the customer's *expectations* before purchasing, the process the customer goes through in making the purchase (in the case of therapy, of securing a service), and the customer's evaluation *after* purchasing. In mental health, the clinician is part of the "product" being purchased, but quality of service will be gauged by many things that have nothing to do with the therapy itself (Morrison, 1996). It is important to keep in mind the distinction between measuring outcome and measuring customer satisfaction. Satisfaction measures may have limited meaning when gathered on an individual provider or on a whole system of care, such as a managed care company. Managed care organizations need to keep their enrolled employers and their employees happy or satisfied. Many will gather enough data to support their position. For example, Samual Mayhugh, the President and CEO of BEHAVIO-RALCARE reported, "Approximately 95% of BEHAVIORALCARE patients report satisfaction with the administrative systems, case management personnel, and providers. An equal percentage of providers report satisfaction with the care management process. Eighty-nine percent of patients report positive posttreatment outcomes" (1996, p. 324). The positive results, as well as other satisfaction findings, are based on expectancies of the patients that are usually fulfilled, but rarely are the expectations compared with alternatives. Nonetheless, managed care organizations and the employers purchasing mental health plans need to be concerned with image and should be concerned that there not be an overt decline in satisfaction, services, or quality. Because mental health services enhance morale and productivity of workers and their families, employers will look to satisfaction data to avoid problems in their benefit packages. "Happy consumers" are likely to stay within a particular managed care system. Consequently, the patient satisfaction information becomes significant.

DOCUMENTING WHAT THE PSYCHOLOGIST DOES IN PRACTICE

One of the strongest recommendations we have for the clinician is to "know thy practice." All too often, we find that clinicians have only vague overall conceptions of the type of practice in which they are engaged. That is, they know the diagnoses and treatment plans for the clients currently being seen, but rarely have a wider perspective on the types of clients seen over a period of a year or longer, their averages and ranges of ages, the diagnoses at presentation, the average number of sessions, the types of interventions employed, the outcomes of the therapy, etc.

The Model Programs project on service delivery programs of the Section on Clinical Child Psychology and the Division of Child, Youth, and Family Services found many exemplary programs that gathered information on their clientele, assessment and treatment actions, client satisfaction, and treatment effectiveness outcome (see Roberts, 1994, 1996). Of the common characteristics of the model programs, a prime one was that they responded to a need for accountability and provided documentation of effectiveness. The programs used the information for purposes of clinical decision-making, component and process analysis, and program evaluation. Empirical documentation is inevitably imperfect, so a variety of data-gathering procedures can demonstrate different aspects of the programs (Roberts & Hinton-Nelson, 1996).

As noted in a previous section, Dr. Carolyn Schroeder has consistently gathered useful data on the pediatric psychology practice attached to the Chapel Hill Pediatrics group in North Carolina (Schroeder, 1996; Schroeder et al., 1983; Schroeder & Gordon, 1991). Program evaluations and fact-based descriptions of the clinical service were incorporated into the database of the business and clinical record-keeping. Dr. Schroeder provides details on the percentages of parental concerns about their children in 22 categories. Additionally, data from the practice and parent questionnaires were analyzed as a function of the age of the child. The average number of visits for clients were also calculated. For example, the median number of visits by presenting problem was computed (e.g., negative behavior: 6 visits; anxiety: 6 visits; learning disability: 4 visits; school problems: 3 visits; divorce/separation: 6 visits; child abuse: 11 visits). These averages compare favorably with industry estimates that 50% of mental health clients are seen for 8 or fewer visits. Many useful pieces of information may be gleaned from the various presentations of the Schroeder practice, including:

- Children appear for certain problems at one age and may reappear in the practice at a later age for a different problem.
- Behavioral interventions can be effective and kept within the typical limitations on numbers of sessions of managed care.

Another example of analyzing diagnostic and therapeutic contacts was described for an adolescent outpatient clinic by Tolan, Ryan, and Jaffe (1988). This clinic had a predominant psychoanalytic orientation. The data bank allowed the clinicians to analyze the use patterns of clinic services (e.g., whether the client returned following intake, dropout stage, total number of contacts) according to client characteristics (e.g., sex, age, ethnic group, complaint type, and DSM-III diagnosis), referral sources, method of payment, and service provider characteristics. Databased descriptions of clinical services can also be found for:

- A behavioral pediatrics clinic in an HMO (Charlop et al., 1987)
- A school system mental health center (Hannah & Nichol, 1996; Paavola, Hannah, & Nichol, 1989)
- Outpatient pediatric and clinical child psychology services (Ottinger & Roberts, 1980; Roberts & Walker, 1989b; Walker, 1979)
- A comprehensive, fully integrated continuum of mental health care (Behar et al., 1996)
- Intensive in-home family preservation programs (Haapala, 1996; Lutzker, 1996)
- Psychological consultation for pediatric rehabilitation (Singer & Drotar, 1989) and services for children with special health care needs (Krahn, Eisert, & Field, 1990)
- A pediatric psychology consultation-liaison service (Olson et al., 1988; Olson & Netherton, 1996)

Dr. Paul Clement (1994, 1996), a California psychologist, offered a quantitative evaluation of his 26 years of private practice. His retrospective file analysis was made possible by nearly complete information that was systematically gathered (and noting frustration when some pieces were not present). He analyzed the relationship of therapy outcome with the types of diagnostic categories and the ages and gender of the clients and presented data on the number of sessions (median average = 12), types of treatments (19 different types used), and referral sources (e.g., other psychologist: 30.8%; physician: 12.5%; managed care company: 8.9%). Clement's analysis was for cases mostly seen before the rise of managed care, but he notes that most of his cases were treated within the session limits typically imposed by these companies. Based on his experience he offers four recommendations to practitioners:

1	The clinician should replicate his analysis on the clinician's own practice to add useful information for other practitioners.
2	The clinician should try to provide the most therapeutic impact in a few sessions.
3	The clinician should evaluate his or her procedures and outcomes in order to refine the practice to be more efficient and effective through self-evaluation.
4	The clinician should determine the referral sources for the practice so that a personal marketing plan can be devised.

Clement notes that only by the clinician's emphasis on *documenting* quality of care can quality be achieved. The clinician can then focus on the diagnostic groups, age groups, or other characteristics for which the best results are obtained, while referring to other clinicians for treatment of less optimal situations for the clinician.

We think that clinicians should become self-researchers, perhaps in ways not taught in graduate school, in order to know their own practices and document what they do and how they do it. By systematic gathering of data on their practices, clinicians can have materials ready for application to managed care panels. Recently, the business manager for a child psychology practice made a bid to subcontract child and family services for a capitated behavioral health plan in a local area. The bid was successful, in her view, because the clinicians in the practice had, from the very beginning, gathered data on their clients as well as the number and types of diagnostic assessments and therapeutic interventions. They could easily demonstrate that the average number of treatment sessions was below the typical number of sessions approved by the plan, that the types of problems presenting in this population were amenable to the types of interventions employed by these clinicians, and that there was a high level of parent and referral source satisfaction. Telephone or mail follow-up requesting information about amelioration of symptoms was also standard practice. This documentation was even more convincing because the numbers were generated without the regulation of a managed care company to keep numbers of sessions down. The business manager believed that the strong database, especially the average number of treatment sessions, also gained the practice greater credibility and success when appealing for more sessions.

When applying to one managed care plan, another clinician was requested to provide documentation on average number of sessions, the types of interventions used for specified types of presenting problems, and parent satisfaction with services. A quick chart review was conducted to provide the information on sessions and problems/interventions, but no retrospective sampling of consumer satisfaction could be conducted quickly. Consequently, we suggest clinicians take a proactive stance to gathering basic information on practice parameters.

Epilogue

In this book, we have provided an overview of issues relevant to child clinicians and others concerned with clinical practice in a managed care environment. It is our belief that managed care can be a minefield through which everybody must step carefully in order for clinicians to provide and patients to receive quality services. We have reviewed several relevant legal and ethical concerns, with the ongoing caveat to consult an attorney before committing to any legally binding arrangements and whenever the clinician is unsure of the implications of procedures, contracts, relationships, or state and federal laws.

We have discussed ways we believe clinicians can perform ethically and competently in a managed care environment while protecting their practice and professional independence as much as possible. These approaches will require at least some modifications in current business practices. The clinician will need to recognize that he or she may sometimes turn down a contract that promises to be lucrative because it violates the clinician's professionalism. We have provided supporting information and documents to help the clinician make justifiable decisions regarding managed care procedures and his or her own practice.

For those clinicians who choose not to accept managed care contracts, we have provided several options for expanding their businesses into other untapped markets. It is our sincere hope that the readers of this volume will find the information herein helpful and even inspirational in the provision of accessible and high-quality services to children and families.

Managed care is entering into a new generation—one in which the cost-containment strategies such as restriction of services will not be acceptable (nor profitable, as most of the potential cost savings will have already been taken). The new generation will be one in which public demands for quality services, accessibility, and accountability will enhance the position of the competent psychologist specializing in children, adolescents, and families. Managed care can recognize this need for change and achieve it on its own because of its own self-interests. As managed care companies strive for an edge in a competitive arena, they will have to truly innovate to find better ways of doing business. This will mean not just paying lip service to "providing" a range of specialty services and not just touting "quality of care" concepts, but actually providing them. This should be the future. If not, then the move toward greater regulation at the federal and state levels brought about by public/consumer outcry and litigation will force changes more in the direction of quality in care.

References

Allen, J. S., Tarnowski, K. J., Simonian, S. J., Elliott, D., & Drabman, R. S. (1991). The generalization map revisited: Assessment of generalized treatment effects in child and adolescent behavior therapy. *Behavior Therapy, 22,* 393–405.

American Medical Association. (1996). *Physicians' current procedural terminology.* Chicago: Author.

American Psychological Association. (1992). Ethical principles of psychologists and code of conduct. *American Psychologist, 47,* 1597–1611.

American Psychological Association Practice Directorate. (1996, June). *The Committee for the Advancement of Professional Practice (CAPP) practitioner survey results.* Washington, DC: Author.

Appelbaum, P. S. (1993). Legal liability and managed care. *American Psychologist, 48,* 251–257.

Armenti, N. P. (1991). The provider network in managed care. *The Behavior Therapist, 14,* 123–126, 128.

Armenti, N. P. (1993). Managed mental health care and the behaviorally trained professional. *The Behavior Therapist, 16,* 13–15.

Austad, C. S., & Hoyt, M. F. (1992). The managed care movement and the future of psychotherapy. *Psychotherapy, 29,* 109–118.

Barkley, R. A. (1991). *Attention-deficit hyperactivity disorder: A clinical workbook.* New York: Guilford.

Behar, L., Bickman, L., Lane, T., Keeton, W. P., Schwartz, M., & Brannock, J. E. (1996). The Fort Bragg child and adolescent mental health demonstration project. In M. C. Roberts (Ed.), *Model programs in child and family mental health* (pp. 351–372). Mahwah, NJ: Erlbaum.

Bennett, M. J., & Gavalya, A. S. (1982). Prepaid comprehensive mental health services for children. *Journal of the American Academy of Psychiatry, 21,* 486–491.

Bickman, L., Guthrie, P. R., Foster, E. M., Lambert, E. W., Summerfelt, W. T., Breda, C. S., & Heflinger, C. A. (1995). *Evaluating managed mental health services: The Fort Bragg experiment.* New York: Plenum.

Bittker, T. E., & Idzorek, S. (1978). The evolution of psychiatric services in a health maintenance organization. *American Journal of Psychiatry, 135,* 339–342.

Borenstein, D. B. (1990). Managed care: A means of rationing psychiatric treatment. *Hospital and Community Psychiatry, 41,* 1095–1098.

Bowers, T. G., & Knapp, S. (1993). Reimbursement issues for psychologists in independent practice. *Psychotherapy in Private Practice, 12,* 73–87.

Brady, J., & Krizay, J. (1985). Utilization and coverage of mental health services in health maintenance organizations. *American Journal of Psychiatry, 142,* 744–746.

Broskowski, A. (1991). Current mental health care environment: Why managed care is necessary. *Professional Psychology: Research and Practice, 22,* 6–14.

Browning, C. H., & Browning, B. J. (1996). *How to partner with managed care.* New York: Wiley.

BT survey results: The changing mental healthcare delivery system. (1987, July 20). *Behavior Today,* pp. 1–2.

Calvert, S. C., & Johnston, C. (1990). Acceptability of treatments for child behavior problems: Issues and implications for future research. *Journal of Clinical Child Psychology, 19,* 61–74.

Cantor, D. W. (1997, January). Open letter to managed care. *APA Monitor,* 2.

Carr, B. (1996, September). Seize the opportunity in primary healthcare setting. *Texas Psychological Association Newsletter, 5,* 10–12.

Casey, R. J., & Berman, J. S. (1985). The outcome of psychotherapy with children. *Psychological Bulletin, 98,* 388–400.

Charlop, M. H., Parrish, J. M., Fenton, L. R., & Cataldo, M. F. (1987). Evaluation of hospital-based outpatient pediatric psychology services. *Journal of Pediatric Psychology, 12,* 485–503.

Christophersen, E. R. (1994). *Pediatric compliance: A guide for the primary care physician.* New York: Plenum Medical.

Church, G. J. (1997, April 14). Backlash against HMOs. *Time,* 32–36.

Clement, P. W. (1994). Quantitative evaluation of 26 years of private practice. *Professional Psychology: Research and Practice, 25,* 173–176.

Clement, P. W. (1996). Evaluation in private practice. *Clinical Psychology: Science and Practice, 3,* 146–159.

Consumers Union. (1995, November). Mental health: Does therapy help? *Consumer Reports,* 734–739.

Consumers Union. (1996, August). How good is your health plan? *Consumer Reports,* 28–42.

Cummings, N. (1995). Impact of managed care on employment and training: A primer for survival. *Professional Psychology: Research and Practice, 26,* 10–15.

Cummings, N. (1996, November). A conversation with Nick Cummings: Now we're facing the consequences. *The Scientist Practitioner, 6*(1), 9–13.

Cummings, N. A., & Follette, W. T. (1968). Psychiatric services and medical utilization in a prepaid health plan setting: Part II. *Medical Care, 6,* 31–41.

Diaz, C., Starfield, B., Holtzman, N., Mellits, E. D., Hankin, J., Smalky, K., & Benson, P. (1986). Ill health and use of medical care: Community-based assessment of morbidity in children. *Medical Care, 24,* 848–856.

Dorwart, R. A. (1990). Managed mental health care: Myths and realities in the 1990s. *Hospital and Community Psychiatry, 41,* 1087–1091.

Drotar, D. (1995). *Consulting with pediatricians: Psychological perspectives.* New York: Plenum.

Durlak, J. A., Fuhrman, T., & Lampman, C. (1991). Effectiveness of cognitive-behavior therapy for maladapting children: A meta-analysis. *Psychological Bulletin, 110,* 204–214.

Employee Retirement Income Security Act of 1974, 29 U. S. C. Section 1143 (1982).

Eyberg, S. M., & Ross, A. W. (1978). Assessment of child behavior problems: The validation of a new inventory. *Journal of Clinical Child Psychology, 7,* 113–116.

Eysenck, H. J. (1952). The effects of psychotherapy: An evaluation. *Journal of Consulting Psychology, 16,* 319–324.

Fee, practice, and managed care survey. (1995, January). *Psychotherapy Finances,* 1–8.

Feldman, J. M., & Kazdin, A. E. (1995). Parent management training for oppositional and conduct problem children. *The Clinical Psychologist, 48*(4), 3–5.

Finney, J. W., Lemanek, K. L., Cataldo, M. F., Katz, H. P., & Fuqua, R. W. (1989). Pediatric psychology in primary health care: Brief targeted therapy for recurrent abdominal pain. *Behavior Therapy, 20,* 283–291.

Finney, J. W., Riley, A. W., & Cataldo, M. F. (1991). Psychology in primary health care: Effects of brief targeted therapy on children's medical care utilization. *Journal of Pediatric Psychology, 16,* 447–461.

Forehand, R. L., & McMahon, R. J. (1981). *Helping the noncompliant child: A clinician's guide to parent training.* New York: Guilford.

Fox, R. E. (1989). Proceedings of the American Psychological Association, Incorporated, for the Year 1988. *American Psychologist, 44,* 996–1028.

Fox, R. E. (1995). The rape of psychotherapy. *Professional Psychology: Research and Practice, 26,* 147–155.

Fraser, J. S. (1996). All that glitters is not always gold: Medical offset effects and managed behavioral health care. *Professional Psychology: Research and Practice, 27,* 335–344.

Friedman, R. M., & Kutash, K. (1992). Challenges for child and adolescent mental health. *Health Affairs, 11,* 125–136.

Friedman, R., Sobel, D., Myers, P., Caudill, M., & Benson, H. (1995). Behavioral medicine, clinical health psychology, and cost offset. *Health Psychology, 14,* 509–518.

Garland, A. F., & Besinger, B. A. (1996). Adolescents' perceptions of outpatient mental health services. *Journal of Child and Family Studies, 5,* 355–375.

Giles, T. R. (1993). *Managed mental health care: A guide for practitioners, employers, and hospital administrators.* Boston: Allyn and Bacon.

Giolas, D. (1996). Computerized treatment planning: Toward interoperable systems. In C. Stout (Ed.), *The complete guide to managed behavioral healthcare* (No. IV, pp. D.1–12). New York: Wiley.

Gordon, B. N., & Schroeder, C. S. (1995). *Sexuality.* New York: Plenum.

Graves, R. L., & Hastrup, J. L. (1981). Psychological intervention and medical utilization in children and adolescents of low-income families. *Professional Psychology, 12,* 426–433.

Groth-Marnat, G., & Edkins, G. (1996). Professional psychologists in general health care settings: A review of the financial efficacy of direct treatment interventions. *Professional Psychology: Research and Practice, 27,* 161–174.

Haapala, D. A. (1996). The Homebuilders model: An evolving service approach for families. In M. C. Roberts (Ed.), *Model programs in child and family mental health* (pp. 295–315). Mahwah, NJ: Erlbaum.

Hankin, J. R., Starfield, B. H., Steinwachs, D. M., Benson, P., Livingston, G., & Katz, H. P. (1984). The relationship between specialized mental health care and patterns of primary care use among children enrolled in a prepaid group practice. *Research in Community Mental Health, 4,* 203–230.

Hannah, F. P., & Nichol, G. T. (1996). Memphis City Schools mental health center. In M. C. Roberts (Ed.), *Model programs in child and family mental health* (pp. 173–192). Mahwah, NJ: Erlbaum.

Hazelrigg, M. D., Cooper, H. M., & Borduin, C. M. (1987). Evaluating the effectiveness of family therapies: An integrative review and analysis. *Psychological Bulletin, 101,* 428–442.

Health insurance inflation stays low—for now. (1997, January 21). *The Kansas City Star,* D-6.

Health Maintenance Organization Act of 1973, 42 U. S. C. Sections 280 (c), 300 (e)(1)(d), 300 (e)(1)(b). (1987).

Hembree-Kigin, T., & McNeil, C. B. (1995). *Parent–child interaction therapy.* New York: Plenum.

Hersch, L. (1995). Adapting to healthcare reform and managed care: Three strategies for survival and growth. *Professional Psychology: Research and Practice, 26,* 16–26.

Hibbs, E. D., & Jensen, P. S. (Eds.). (1996). *Psychosocial treatments for child and adolescent disorders: Empirically based strategies for clinical practice.* Washington, DC: American Psychological Association.

Higuchi, S. A. (1994). Recent managed-care legislative and legal issues. In R. L. Lowman & R. J. Resnick (Eds.), *The mental health professional's guide to managed care* (pp. 83–118). Washington, DC: American Psychological Association.

Homchick, R. G. (1994, February 28). Come together, right now. *Legal Times*, 7.

Houts, A. C. (1996). Behavioral treatment of enuresis. *The Clinical Psychologist, 49*(1), 5–6.

Howard, K. I., Lueger, R. J., Maling, M. S., & Martinovich, Z. (1993). A phase model of psychotherapy outcome: Causal mediation of change. *Journal of Consulting and Clinical Psychology, 61*, 678–685.

Hurley, L. K. (1995). Developing a collaborative pediatric psychology practice in a pediatric primary care setting. In D. Drotar, *Consulting with pediatricians: Psychological perspectives* (pp. 159–171). New York: Plenum.

Jacobson, N. S., Follette, W. C., & Revenstorf, D. (1986). Toward a standard definition of clinically significant change. *Behavior Therapy, 17*, 308–311.

Kazdin, A. E. (1988). *Child psychotherapy: Developing and identifying effective treatments.* Elmsford, NY: Pergamon.

Kazdin, A. E. (1993). Psychotherapy for children and adolescents: Current progress and future research directions. *American Psychologist, 48*, 644–657.

Kazdin, A. E. (1996). Evaluation in clinical practice—Introduction to the series. *Clinical Psychology: Science and Practice, 3*, 144–145.

Kazdin, A. E., Bass, D., Ayers, W. A., & Rodgers, A. (1990). Empirical and clinical focus of child and adolescent psychotherapy research. *Journal of Consulting and Clinical Psychology, 60*, 733–747.

Kazdin, A. E., French, N., & Sherick, R. (1981). Acceptability of alternative treatments for children: Evaluations by inpatient children, parents, and staff. *Journal of Consulting and Clinical Psychology, 49*, 900–907.

Kearney, J. R. (1995, May 8). Dear Colleague letter. The Kansas Institute, Shawnee Mission, Kansas.

Kelleher, K., & Starfield, B. (1990). Health care use by children receiving mental health services. *Pediatrics, 85*, 114–118.

Kiresuk, T. J., & Sherman, R. E. (1968). Goal attainment scaling: A general method for evaluating comprehensive community mental health programs. *Community Mental Health Journal, 4*, 443–453.

Klett, A. L., & Rashap, J. L. (1996). Parent–child interaction therapy: Training to meet the needs of the 21st century. *The Behavior Therapist, 19*, 120–121.

Knitzer, J. (1982). *Unclaimed children: The failure of public responsibility to children and adolescents in need of mental health services.* Washington, DC: Children's Defense Fund.

Knitzer, J. (1993). Children's mental health policy: Challenging the future. *Journal of Emotional and Behavioral Disorders, 1*, 8–16.

Kovacs, M. (1981). Rating scales to assess depression in school-aged children. *Acta Paedopsychiatrica, 46*, 305–315.

Krahn, G. L., Eisert, D., & Fifield, B. (1990). Obtaining parental perceptions of the quality of services for children with special health needs. *Journal of Pediatric Psychology, 15*, 761–774.

Lambert, M. J., & Brown, G. S. (1996). Data-based management for tracking outcome in private practice. *Clinical Psychology: Science and Practice, 3*, 172–178.

Levinson, J. C. (1993). *Guerrilla marketing.* New York: Houghton Mifflin.

Levinson, J. C., & Godin, S. (1994). *The guerrilla marketing handbook.* New York: Houghton Mifflin.

Levitt, E. E. (1957). The results of psychotherapy with children: An evaluation. *Journal of Consulting Psychology, 32*, 286–289.

Levitt, E. E. (1963). Psychotherapy with children: A further evaluation. *Behavior Research and Therapy, 60*, 326–329.

Lipsey, M. W., & Wilson, D. B. (1993). The efficacy of psychological, educational, and behavioral treatment: Confirmation from meta-analysis. *American Psychologist, 48,* 1191–1209.

Ludwigsen, J. R., & Enright, M. F. (1988). The health care revolution: Implications for psychology and hospital practice. *Psychotherapy, 25,* 424–428.

Lutzker, J. R. (1996). An ecobehavioral model for serious family disorders: Child abuse and neglect; developmental disabilities. In M. C. Roberts (Ed.), *Model programs in child and family mental health* (pp. 33–46). Mahwah, NJ: Erlbaum.

Managed care: 10 areas to check before signing contracts. (1994, July). *Psychotherapy Finances, 6.*

Mangan, D. (1993, June 14). Is this the salvation of private practice? *Medical Economics,* 146–156.

Mash, E. J., & Hunsley, J. (1993). Behavior therapy and managed mental health care: Integrating effectiveness and economics in mental health practice. *Behavior Therapy, 24,* 67–90.

Matson, J. L. (Ed.). (1988). *Handbook of treatment approaches in childhood psychopathology.* New York: Plenum.

Mayhugh, S. (1996). Managed care: Strongly conflicting views. *Professional Psychology: Research and Practice, 27,* 323–324.

McCann, D. C. (1996, November). Practical suggestions for keeping afloat in private mental health care practice. *Texas Psychological Association Newsletter,* 6–7.

Miller, I. J. (1996a). National Committee for Quality Assurance (NCQA): Who is the watchdog's master? *The Independent Practitioner, 16,* 133–137.

Miller, I. J. (1996b). Managed care is harmful to outpatient mental health services: A call for accountability. *Professional Psychology: Research and Practice, 27,* 349–363.

Miller, R. H., & Luft, H. S. (1994). Managed care plan performance since 1980: A literature analysis. *Journal of the American Medical Association, 271,* 1512–1519.

Morrison, D. (1996). Treating patients as customers. In C. Stout (Ed.), *The complete guide to managed behavioral healthcare* (No. II, pp. A.3–11). New York: Wiley.

Mumford, E., Schlesinger, H. J., Glass, G. V., Patrick, C., & Cuerdon, T. (1984). A new look at evidence about reduced cost of medical utilization following mental health treatment. *American Journal of Psychiatry, 141,* 1145–1158.

New anti-trust guidelines issued by federal agencies showed greater tolerance of provider networks. (1996, October). *Psychotherapy Finances* Website: http://www.psyfin.com/psyfin/oct96/antitrust.htm.

New Jersey psychologists file precedent-setting lawsuit against managed care company. (1996, August). *Kansas Psychologist, 22*(3), 11–12.

Newman, R. (1995, March). Legal tack could ease managed-care woes. *APA Monitor,* 32.

Newman, R., & Bricklin, P. M. (1991). Parameters of managed mental health care: Legal, ethical, and professional guidelines. *Professional Psychology: Research and Practice, 22,* 26–35.

O'Hara, M. (1996). Divided we stand. *The Family Therapy Networker, 20*(5), 46–53.

Ollendick, T. H., King, N. J., & Yule, W. (Eds.). (1994). *International handbook of phobic and anxiety disorders in children and adolescents.* New York: Plenum.

Olson, R. A., Holden, E. W., Friedman, A., Faust, J., Kenning, M., & Mason, P. J. (1988). Psychological consultation in a children's hospital: An evaluation of services. *Journal of Pediatric Psychology, 13,* 479–492.

Olson, R., & Netherton, S. D. (1996). Consultation and liaison in a children's hospital. In M. C. Roberts (Ed.), *Model programs in child and family mental health* (pp. 249–264). Mahwah, NJ: Erlbaum.

Ottinger, D. R., & Roberts, M. C. (1980). A university-based predoctoral program in pediatric psychology. *Professional Psychology, 11,* 707–713.

Paavola, J. C., Hannah, F. P., & Nichol, G. T. (1989). The Memphis City Schools Mental Health Center: A program description. *Professional School Psychology, 4,* 61–74.

Padgett, D. K., Patrick, C., Burns, B. J., Schlesinger, H. J., & Cohen, J. (1993). The effect of insurance benefit changes on use of child and adolescent outpatient mental health services. *Medical Care, 31,* 96–110.

Parloff, M. B. (1984). Psychotherapy research and its incredible credibility crisis. *Clinical Psychology Review, 4,* 95–109.

Paul, G. L. (1967). Outcome research in psychotherapy. *Journal of Consulting Psychology, 31,* 109–118.

Pelham, W. E., Greiner, A. R., Gnagy, E. M., Hoza, B., Martin, L., Sams, S. E., & Wilson, T. (1996). Intensive treatment for ADHD: A model summer treatment program. In M. C. Roberts (Ed.), *Model programs in child and family mental health* (pp. 193–213). Mahwah, NJ: Erlbaum.

Pelham, W. E., & Hoza, B. (1996). Intensive treatment: A summer treatment program for children with ADHD. In E. D. Hibbs & P. S. Jensen (Eds.), *Psychosocial treatment of child and adolescent disorders: Empirically based strategies for clinical practice* (pp. 311–340). Washington, DC: American Psychological Association.

Perrott, L. A. (1996, Fall). It's the paradigm, stupid! *The Independent Practitioner, 16,* 193–196.

Peterson, L., & Harbeck, C. (1988). *The pediatric psychologist.* Champaign, IL: Research Press.

Pfander, S., & Seagull, E. A. (1992). The effect of pediatric psychologic consultation on the management of adolescent suicide attempts in the pediatric service of a general hospital. *American Journal of Diseases of Children, 146,* 898–900.

Pfeiffer, S. I., & Shott, S. (1996). Treatment outcomes assessment: Conceptual, practical, and ethical considerations. In C. Stout (Ed.), *The complete guide to managed behavioral healthcare* (No. II, pp. E.1–11). New York: Wiley.

Pollard, M., & Tilson, H. H. (1996). Legal and regulatory issues in managed behavioral healthcare. In C. Stout (Ed.), *The complete guide to managed behavioral healthcare* (No. III., pp. B.3–11). New York: Wiley.

Practitioner survey results offer comprehensive view of psychology practice. (1996, June). *Practitioner Update, 4*(2), 1–5.

Rae, W. A. (1987). We must change our approach to psychosocial care: Fitting the pan to the ham. *Children's Health Care, 15,* 216–217.

Resnick, R. J., Bottinelli, R. W., Puder-York, M., Harris, B., & O'Keefe, B. E. (1994). Basic issues in managed mental health services. In R. L. Lowman & Resnick, R. J. (Eds.), *The mental health professional's guide to managed care* (pp. 41–62). Washington, DC: American Psychological Association.

Reynolds, W. M., & Johnston, H. F. (Eds.). (1994). *Handbook of depression in children and adolescents.* New York: Plenum.

Richardson, L. M., & Austad, C. S. (1991). Realities of mental health practice in managed care settings. *Professional Psychology: Research and Practice, 22,* 52–59.

Roberts, M. C. (1986). *Pediatric psychology.* New York: Pergamon.

Roberts, M. C. (1994). Models for service delivery in children's mental health: Common characteristics. *Journal of Clinical Child Psychology, 23,* 212–219.

Roberts, M. C. (Ed.). (1995). *Handbook of pediatric psychology* (2nd ed.). New York: Guilford.

Roberts, M. C. (Ed.). (1996). *Model programs in child and family mental health.* Mahwah, NJ: Erlbaum.

Roberts, M. C., Carlson, C. I., Erickson, M. T., Friedman, R. M., La Greca, A. M., Lemanek, K. L., Russ, S. W., Schroeder, C. S., Vargas, L. A., & Wohlford, P. F. (submitted). A model for training psychologists to provide services for children and adolescents.

Roberts, M. C., Erickson, M. T., & Tuma, J. M. (1985). Addressing the needs: Guidelines for training psychologists to work with children, youth, and families. *Journal of Clinical Child Psychology, 14,* 70–79.

Roberts, M. C., & Hinton-Nelson, M. (1996). Models for service delivery in child and family mental health. In M. C. Roberts (Ed.), *Model programs in child and family mental health* (pp. 1–21). Mahwah, NJ: Erlbaum.

Roberts, M. C., & Walker, C. E. (Eds.). (1989a). *Casebook of child and pediatric psychology.* New York: Guilford.

Roberts, M. C., & Walker, C. E. (1989b). Clinical cases in child and pediatric psychology: Conceptualization and overview. In M. C. Roberts & C. E. Walker (Eds.), *Casebook of child and pediatric psychology* (pp. 1–15). New York: Guilford.

Roberts, M. C., & Wright, L. (1982). The role of the pediatric psychologist as consultant to pediatricians. In J. M. Tuma (Ed.), *Handbook for the practice of pediatric psychology* (pp. 251–289). New York: Wiley.

Rodrigue, J. R., Hoffman, R. G., Rayfield, A., Lescano, C., Kubar, W., Streisand, R., & Banko, C. (1995). Evaluating pediatric psychology consultation services in a medical setting: An example. *Journal of Clinical Psychology in Medical Settings, 2,* 89–107.

Rosen, J. C., & Wiens, A. N. (1979). Changes in medical problems and use of medical services following psychological intervention. *American Psychologist, 34,* 420–431.

Saxe, L., Cross, T., & Silverman, N. (1988). Children's mental health: The gap between what we know and what we do. *American Psychologist, 43,* 800–807.

Schachner, M. (1994, January 10). Mental health group practices on the rise. *Business Insurance, 3,* 36.

Schroeder, C. S. (1996). Mental health services in pediatric primary care. In M. C. Roberts (Ed.), *Model programs in child and family mental health* (pp. 265–284). Mahwah, NJ: Erlbaum.

Schroeder, C. S., & Gordon, B. N. (1991). *Assessment and treatment of childhood problems.* New York: Guilford.

Schroeder, C. S., Gordon, B. N., Kanoy, K., & Routh, D. K. (1983). Managing children's behavior problems in pediatric practice. In M. Wolraich & D. K. Routh (Eds.), *Advances in developmental and behavioral pediatrics* (Vol. 4, pp. 25–86). Greenwich, CT: JAI Press.

Seligman, M. E. P. (1995). The effectiveness of psychotherapy: The *Consumer Reports* study. *American Psychologist, 50,* 965–974.

Seligman, M. E. P. (1996). The pitfalls of managed care. *Kansas Psychologist, 22*(3), 6, 8.

Shirk, S. R., & Phillips, J. S. (1991). Child therapy training: Closing gaps with research and practice. *Journal of Consulting and Clinical Psychology, 59,* 766–776.

Shirk, S. R., & Russell, R. L. (1992). A reevaluation of estimates of child therapy effectiveness. *Journal of the American Academy of Child and Adolescent Psychiatry, 31,* 703–709.

Shore, K. (1996). An alternative view: Comments of Karen Shore. *Professional Psychology: Research and Practice, 27,* 324.

Shulman, M. E. (1988). Cost containment in clinical psychology: Critique of Biodyne and the HMOs. *Professional Psychology: Research and Practice, 19,* 298–307.

Sikorszky, R. (1996). Treatment planning and automated assistance—Update 1. In C. Stout (Ed.), *The complete guide to managed behavioral healthcare* (No. IV, pp. C.1–13). New York: Wiley.

Silverman, W. K., & Kurtines, W. M. (1996). *Anxiety and phobic disorders: A pragmatic approach.* New York: Plenum.

Singer, L., & Drotar, D. (1989). Psychological practice in a pediatric rehabilitation hospital. *Journal of Pediatric Psychology, 14,* 479–489.

Sinnett, E. R., & Holen, M. C. (1993). The perceived influence of health insurance on psychological services. *Psychotherapy in Private Practice, 12,* 41–50.

Sleek, S. (1995, July). Company alters rule on providers' public complaints. *APA Monitor,* 41.

Sleek, S. (1996a, October). APA's efforts key to securing parity for mental health. *APA Monitor,* 7.

Sleek, S. (1996b, November). State laws are reining in managed care. *APA Monitor,* 1, 34.

Sleek, S. (1996c, November). State legislation aims to boost patient protections. *APA Monitor*, 34.

Sleek, S. (1996d, December). Psychology continues its call for equity. *APA Monitor*, 28, 30.

Sleek, S. (1997, February). Managed care: The new media bad guy. *APA Monitor*, 30.

Smith, M. L., & Glass, G. V. (1977). Meta-analysis of psychotherapy outcome studies. *American Psychologist, 32*, 752–760.

Sobel, D. S. (1994). Mind matters, money matters: The cost-effectiveness of clinical behavioral medicine. In *New research frontiers in behavioral medicine: Proceedings of the National Conference* (NIH Publication No. 94-3772; pp. 25–36). Washington, DC: Government Printing Office.

Special report: Increasing your self-pay practice in an era of managed care. (1996). *Psychotherapy Finances,* 1–16.

Strupp, H. (1996). The tripartite model and the *Consumer Reports* study. *The American Psychologist, 51*, 1017–1024.

Sullivan, M. J. (1996, August.) Rhode Island psychologists build connections with the business community. *Practitioner Focus, 9*(1), 9.

Takayama, J. I., Bergman, A. B., & Connell, F. A. (1994). Children in foster care in the state of Washington: Health care utilization and expenditures. *Journal of the American Medical Association, 271*, 1850–1855.

Task Force on Promotion and Dissemination of Psychological Procedures, Division of Clinical Psychology, American Psychological Association. (1995). Training in and dissemination of empirically-validated psychological treatments: Report and recommendations. *The Clinical Psychologist, 48*(1), 3–23.

Therapy groups: 7 helpful hints for starting profitable groups. (1996). *Psychotherapy Finances*, (supplement), 8–9.

Todd, D. M., Jacobus, S. I., & Boland, J. (1992). Uses of a computer database to support research-practice integration in a training clinic. *Professional Psychology: Research and Practice, 23*, 52–58.

Tolan, P., Ryan, K., & Jaffe, C. (1988). Adolescents' mental health service use and provider, process, and recipient characteristics. *Journal of Clinical Child Psychology, 17*, 229–236.

Vein, C. A., & Cullen, E. A. (1996). APA influences evolution of NCQA accreditation standards. *Practitioner Focus, 9*(2), 6, 18.

Walker, C. E. (1979). Behavioral intervention in a pediatric setting. In J. R. McNamera (Ed.), *Behavioral approaches to medicine: Applications and analysis* (pp. 227–266). New York: Plenum.

Walker, C. E., & Roberts, M. C. (Eds.). (1992). *Handbook of clinical child psychology* (2nd ed.). New York: Wiley.

Wall, B., Solum, R. S., & Sobol, M. R. (1992). *The visionary leader*. Rocklin, CA: Prima Publishing.

Weisz, J. R., & Weiss, B. (1993). *Effects of psychotherapy with children and adolescents*. Newbury Park, CA: Sage.

Weisz, J. R., Weiss, B., Alicke, M. D., & Klotz, M. L. (1987). Effectiveness of psychotherapy with children and adolescents: A meta-analysis for clinicians. *Journal of Consulting and Clinical Psychology, 55*, 542–549.

Wells, M. G., Burlingame, G. M., Lambert, M. J., Hoag, M. J., & Hope, C. A. (1996). Conceptualization and measurement of patient change during psychotherapy: Development of the Outcome Questionnaire and Youth Outcome Questionnaire. *Psychotherapy, 33*, 275–283.

Wickline v. State of California, 228 Cal. Reptr. 661 (Cal.App. 2 Dist., 1986).

Widmeyer Group, Inc. (1994). *APA member focus groups on the health care environment: A summary report*. Washington, DC: American Psychological Association.

Wiggins, J. G. (1996). Stress, behavioral physiology, capitation, and the future of psychology. *The Independent Practitioner, 16,* 126–128.

Wilkes, T. C. R., Belsher, G., Rush, A. J., & Frank, E. (1994). *Cognitive therapy for depressed adolescents.* New York: Guilford.

Wilson v. Blue Cross of Southern California, 271 Cal. Reptr. 876 (Cal.App. 2 Dist., 1990).

Winegar, N. (1996). *The clinician's guide to managed behavioral care.* New York: Haworth.

Winegar, N., & Bistline, J. L. (1994). *Marketing mental health services to managed care.* New York: Haworth.

Wooley, S. C. (1993). Managed care and mental health: The silencing of a profession. *International Journal of Eating Disorders, 14,* 387–401.

Woolhandler, S., & Himmelstein, D. V. (1996). Annotation: Patients on the auction block. *American Journal of Public Health, 86,* 1699–1700.

Wright, R. (1992). The cons of psychotherapy in managed health care. *Psychotherapy in Private Practice, 11,* 71–77.

Yenney, S. L., & APA Practice Directorate. (1994). *Business strategies for a caring profession.* Washington, DC: American Psychological Association.

Zusman, J. (1990). Utilization review: Theory, practice, and issues. *Hospital and Community Psychiatry, 41,* 531–536.

Index